Treatment of Cerebral Palsy
and Motor Delay

Treatment of Cerebral Palsy and Motor Delay

SOPHIE LEVITT

BSc (Physiotherapy) Rand, FCSP
Consultant paediatric physiotherapist
Tutor on developmental therapy

THIRD EDITION

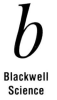

Blackwell
Science

© 1977, 1982, 1995 by Sophie Levitt

Blackwell Science Ltd
Editorial Offices:
Osney Mead, Oxford OX2 0EL
25 John Street, London WC1N 2BL
23 Ainslie Place, Edinburgh EH3 6AJ
350 Main Street, Malden
    MA 02148 5018, USA
54 University Street, Carlton
    Victoria 3053, Australia
10, rue Casimir Delavigne
    75006 Paris, France

Other Editorial Offices:

Blackwell Wissenschafts-Verlag GmbH
Kurfürstendamm 57
10707 Berlin, Germany

Blackwell Science KK
MG Kodenmacho Building
7–10 Kodenmacho Nihombashi
Chuo-ku, Tokyo 104, Japan

First published 1977
Second edition 1982
Reprinted 1983, 1985, 1986, 1987, 1991
Third edition 1995
Reprinted 1996, 1997, 1998, 2000

Set by Best-set Typesetters Ltd, Hong Kong
Printed and bound in the United Kingdom
at the University Press, Cambridge

The Blackwell Science logo is a
trade mark of Blackwell Science Ltd,
registered at the United Kingdom
Trade Marks Registry

DISTRIBUTORS

Marston Book Services Ltd
PO Box 269
Abingdon, Oxon OX14 4YN
(*Orders*: Tel: 01235 465500
            Fax: 01235 465555)

USA
Blackwell Science, Inc.
Commerce Place
350 Main Street
Malden, MA 02148 5018
(*Orders*: Tel: 800 759 6102
            781 388 8250
      Fax: 781 388 8255)

Canada
Login Brothers Book Company
324 Saulteaux Crescent
Winnipeg, Manitoba R3J 3T2
(*Orders*: Tel: 204 837-2987
            Fax: 204 837-3116)

Australia
Blackwell Science Pty Ltd
54 University Street
Carlton, Victoria 3053
(*Orders*: Tel: 03 9347 0300
            Fax: 03 9347 5001)

A catalogue record for this title
is available from the British Library

ISBN 0-632-03873-X

Library of Congress
Cataloging-in-Publication Data

Levitt, Sophie.
    Treatment of cerebral palsy and motor
delay/Sophie Levitt – 3rd ed.
        p.   cm.
    Includes bibliographical references and
index
    ISBN 0–632–03873–X
    1. Cerebal palsied children –
Rehabilitation.   2. Physical therapy for
children.   3. Movement disorders in
children – Treatment.
I. Title.
    [DNLM: 1. Cerebral Palsy –
therapy.   2. Motor Skills.   WS 342
L666t   1994]
RJ496.C4L43   1994
618.92′83603 – dc20
DNLM/DLC
for Library of Congress   94-16798
                                              CIP

For further information on
Blackwell Science, visit our website:
www.blackwell-science.com

Contents

Foreword to Second Edition

Mary D. Sheridan

The happy accident of being a fellow lecturer on a course in developmental paediatrics some years ago brought about my first introduction to Sophie Levitt's work. My attention was immediately engaged by the gentle but firm authority with which she expounded her message to us, an experienced professional audience, and by her well-chosen lantern slides. Later I was impressed by her ease in rapidly establishing good relationships with half a dozen young handicapped children and their mothers who had been called for demonstration, and were previously unknown to her; but above all the lovely competence of her 'laying on of hands' filled me with admiration. Since then I have welcomed any opportunity open to me to see and listen to her in action. No greater compliment than this can be paid by one teacher to another.

She tells us that her aim has been to concentrate on the mechanisms of posture, balance, locomotion and manipulation in normal and physically abnormal children. She discusses how these mechanisms occur, how they are maintained, and how they must be trained to ensure optimum development of mobility and hand skills. But her book covers much wider ground. Experience has taught her the importance of a host of other influences which must be taken into serious consideration in treatment of a child and the counselling of parents. She stresses the importance of a comprehensive assessment which is not mere 'reflex hunting' but takes into account a child's present levels of visual, auditory and language development, his intelligence and personality, and, very importantly the prognosis of his disability. She points out the parents' needs for consistent sympathetic knowledgeable guidance and the necessity for adequate local services for follow-up supervision and education.

Whilst the largest part of her book is devoted to description of, and detailed explanation of, the principles underlying her own therapeutic procedures which she has evolved from wide clinical experience and the selection of some acknowledgeably successful items from numerous previous 'systems', she also provides much helpful advice on other aspects of treatment and training.

The photographs are clear and well-chosen. The drawings are a sheer delight. The book cannot fail to inform and inspire many other workers in the field of developmental paediatrics as it has informed, inspired and indeed comforted me.

Foreword to Third Edition

Brian Neville

Professor of Paediatric Neurology, Institute of Child Health, London
Hon Consultant Paediatric Neurology, Great Ormond Street Hospital
for Children NHS Trust
Chairman of the European Academy of Childhood Disability

It is a great pleasure to welcome the Third Edition of Sophie Levitt's popular book.

The cerebral palsies consist of a group of 'motor' disorders, of infinite variety and severity. Their designation as motor disorders is to some extent arbitrary and a combination of motor, sensory, cognitive and behavioural disability is the common clinical situation. For one hundred years, professionals from different disciplines have tried to shed light on this most difficult group of disorders. In the earlier chapters, the author reviews this litany of famous names with their methods, their classifications and their beliefs in a most helpful and informative way. Her approach, however, is to extract from these sources that which she has found to be helpful in the physical management of motor disabled children. This eclectic approach is clear and throws down the challenge for those who might, for example, insist that a 'normal' developmental sequence should be followed.

The core of this text is a detailed description of the physical management techniques written from the perspective of an experienced therapist with a wide theoretical background. This I believe makes it essential reading for developmental therapists and paediatricians. Having set the scene of this complex subject, the reader is then given a great deal of practical advice on all aspects of physical management. The style of the text is descriptive and problem solving and this makes it easy to use by a clinician with some experience. It does not pretend to deal with the use of orthoses, orthopaedic surgery nor in any detail with the place of modern innovations like rhizotomy and botulinum toxin. The author's energy, enthusiasm and detailed practical and theoretical knowledge of physical therapy is set out in a chapter of 150 pages of excellent text which is illuminated by good line drawings.

The reason for an eclectic approach has to be the limitations in the different methods of physical therapy and particularly in their theoretical basis. Despite some good research in this area, a great deal of the work in this field is likely to remain unsupported by scientific evidence. What are the assumptions underlying the selections that Sophie Levitt has made? I suggest that they are:

(1) Since cure is not achievable, it would be unreasonable for the child and family's life to be totally dominated by physical therapy.
(2) Where possible, prevention of fixed deformity should be a major aim of treatment since it keeps later options open.
(3) Motor progress occurs in sequences of useful gains which need to be flexibly applied. This is a chain of subsidiary aims, not necessarily a neurologically based system.
(4) An eclectic approach in this context is almost inevitably aim orientated (Scrutton 1984).

The clinical issue of any such approach is to whose eclecticism is one referring. Sophie Levitt is describing what she has found useful. She is deliberately not prescribing a new 'system' of her own. This means that readers having been given this invaluable pathway have to make many of their own decisions.

I am sure that the new edition of this book, which draws on many recent publications, deserves a central place in the training and practice of people concerned with the cerebral palsies.

Preface

'What makes a child move?' is a crucial question for those treating cerebral palsied children and children with developmental motor delay. Various answers to this question come from different doctors, physiotherapists, occupational therapists as well as from psychologists and educationalists. In addition those disciplines concerned with deprived social and economic conditions and with the design of environments for handicapped children will offer reasons for limitation of children's movement development through lack of stimulation and motor exploration.

Although recognizing the value of all these ideas, this book is based on the answers given by different doctors, therapists and my own experience. Many workers in this field, in various countries, have generously given me of their time and knowledge. Space does not permit mention of all their names, but they have my deep gratitude. I am particularly appreciative of the privilege of discussions and observations of the work of Dr Phelps, Dr and Mrs Bobath, Dr Fay, Dr Vojta, Miss Knott, Mrs Collis and Dr Hari. They have inspired and influenced me and without them this book could not have been written. Although I have been emotionally drawn to follow each one of them devotedly out of respect for their great contributions, I could not do so. It would have been a denial of my own thoughts and experience, and I hope they will respect this. I have dared to stand on their broad shoulders and attempt to synthesize some of their ideas at this stage of our knowledge.

In working out this synthesis, it has been especially helpful and stimulating to work for many years with Dr John Foley and benefit from his studies and interpretations of Dr Purdon Martin's work in adult and child neurology. I have been encouraged in my eclectic viewpoint not only by Dr Foley and the staff of The Cheyne Centre for Children with Cerebral Palsy, but also by my previous Director, Professor Kenneth Holt, and by the late Professor Robert Collis, by Professor G. Tardieu and many students and colleagues.

My attempts to correlate the neurology of Foley and Purdon Martin to child development depended on the extensive use of the work of the late Dr Mary Sheridan. She is an inspiration to me and many of my colleagues. It is a special honour to have a Foreword by her. I am most grateful.

My experience is also greatly dependent on the parents and children with whom I have been privileged to work and learn so much. It is because of their essential participation that I was unable to write a book 'for therapists only' and the large section on practical procedures (Chapter 7) is divided into Treatment suggestions which can be carried out by both therapists and parents under Daily care. These methods must, however, be *selected* for the child by a physiotherapist and then *shown* to the parents, or to surrogate parents such as nursery nurses, teachers, playgroup workers and others. The others also include speech therapists and occupational therapists who offer their methods to the physiotherapist when indicated. The book includes some of their suggestions.

Parents and therapists
This book takes special account of parents as their cooperation is needed to correctly handle their child throughout the day, sometimes carry out special exercises or manipulations, apply any calipers and use the special aids, correct toys, footwear and other recommendations of therapists. This book, however, does not elaborate on the attitudes of parents which affect the use of the many practical ideas offered. Parents' attitudes are known to affect the progress of their handicapped child. The subject is a vast one as parents are people and the variety of attitudes among people requires much discussion. Many other books have been written on the subject and should be consulted. It is, however, the day-to-day experience of communicating with parents and the advice of various other disciplines working with these parents that will educate the therapist. She must also observe what she does to influence parents' attitudes negatively as well as positively. In summary, the therapist must learn:

- To communicate *to* parents why methods are selected and further explain or repeat what the doctors have said about the child's problems. She must instruct parents in how to do the methods and give them confidence in doing them. She must then have an ongoing supervision of these methods which should be primarily those concerned with the child's daily activities.
- To receive communication *from* parents as to their practical problems and needs, their own suggestions and discoveries, their observations of their child and the questions they really want answered. Receiving communication from parents and the team of workers will also help the therapist put her treatment in a context which is relevant to the child *and* his parents and family. This takes skill so that the parents do not exaggerate their role as 'therapists' to the detriment of the family. Treatment of the handicapped child should not create a handicapped family under severe strain.

The plan of the book
The aim is to present as practical a book as possible as there are already books which review systems of treatment and recommend an open mind, but do not tell the therapist how to *do* it. It is difficult to describe

methods without demonstration. Thus, the therapist should use this book with practical courses, further study, observations and supervision by senior colleagues.

Methods are not in themselves all important. The therapist must know the purpose of each method and if she detects the principle behind it she can invent her own methods besides those suggested in this book. Wherever possible the principle has been given, as to why, when and when not to use methods, but not all possibilities can be covered in a book. Once again, clinical experience and courses are recommended to supplement this book.

The methods have been linked with the problems of the child and rather less with the diagnosis. The causes and the disorders underlying the problem of function are of less concern to therapists and parents and are not given as much prominence in this book. It is the developmental disabilities of motor delay and motor dysfunction which are the problems. These functions are our chief concern. Dr R. MacKeith has said 'we must separate disorder from function' using disorder to mean the underlying signs and symptoms requiring diagnostic procedures.

This Third Edition updates the book with acknowledgement to my reviewers and colleagues who have given me constructive criticism and much encouragement. Since publication of the First and Second Editions there has been an increase in the eclectic viewpoint in the treatment of children with cerebral palsies and motor delay. Recent research and studies have supported my First Edition's views that spasticity, reflex reactions and primitive or pathological responses were overemphasized. Spasticity has more relevance in the genesis of deformities than in directly causing most of the motor disorders or motor dysfunction.

I have been influenced by many approaches on the learning processes involved in developing motor function. As an eclectic worker, I have drawn on different learning methods according to a child's impairments and developmental stages. The learning of parents and carers has interested me particularly as so much depends on their collaboration in enabling their child to develop motor control. Over the years I have therefore drawn on how adults learn in the context of developing a positive relationship with their tutors or therapists. Learning to work together and appreciate the feelings of others is as much part of learning as the cognitive, sensory, perceptual and motor aspects of any motor learning model. For all these reasons the *medical model* in which we physiotherapists are educated has broadened to integrate ideas from psychology, psychotherapy and social work. Thus the diagnostic classifications and neurological labels may not receive the medical emphasis some doctors would prefer. However, many other doctors, aware of the importance of each child's motor function in his or her daily life, have encouraged this shift of emphasis to functional aspects. This book has two new chapters which develop the learning principles from earlier editions and continue my ongoing studies of how to integrate treatment, training and learning in the development of children with motor problems.

Swimming, horse riding, skiing and other recreational activities for the handicapped child are omitted as they are not strictly 'treatment'. They are naturally highly recommended and other publications and films are available in many countries.

It is hoped that this book will respond to some extent to the remarks of my post-graduate students and colleagues who suggested I write it. Remarks such as:

'I agree with your eclectic approach, but how do I go about doing it?'
'How is it possible to combine such different viewpoints in our field?'
'I have followed one system but would like to extend my repertoire of methods.'
'I believe in one system, but am open to hearing other viewpoints.'

but especially to the remark:

'Help me help these children and their families.'

Note: For the sake of clarity, children will be referred to throughout as male and therapists as female. In fact, considering that therapists are more often female and boys are more often handicapped than girls in many conditions, this may be acceptable. The use of 'he' and 'she' will thus be clear and consistent throughout the text.

Sophie Levitt

Acknowledgements

I am grateful to the Leverhulme Trust Fund who kindly awarded me a Research Fellowship for part of my studies on the Synthesis of Treatment Systems in Cerebral Palsy which form the foundation of this book.

This book was commenced when I was Director of Studies at The Cheyne Centre for Children with Cerebral Palsy, and the Centre gave me encouraging support for which I thank them.

With acknowledgements to Dr P.M. Sonksen from her thesis (1978) for MD entitled: *The neurodevelopmental and paediatric findings associated with significant disabilities of language development* (The Wolfson Centre Library, Mecklenburgh Square, London WC1) for Tables 7.2 to 7.5.

Acknowledgement is made for the kind and generous help of the following: Miss Alison Wisbeach OTR for all the drawings. The late Dr Mary Sheridan, late Dr R. MacKeith and the late Professors R. Collis and G. Tardieu. My colleagues with whom I worked at The Cheyne Centre for Children with Cerebral Palsy, The Wolfson Centre and in many countries abroad. Thanks are also due to The Indian Spastics Society (Delhi and Bombay).

I feel priviliged to have been awarded a Folke Bernadotte fellowship supported by the Paediatric group of the Swedish Physiotherapy Association and their chairperson Elisabeth Price in 1990. Their encouragement of my eclectic approach and work with parents has been an inspiration. The honour of being a patron of the New Zealand Home Visiting Therapists from 1985 has also given me support which I value.

My thanks are also due to Dr Joan Reynell, Dr Pam Zinkin, Ms Margaret Black, the late Mary Kitzinger and Dr Patricia Sonksen with whom I worked on severely visually impaired children. Michelle Lee, Alison Wisbeach, Lesley Carroll, Katrin Stroh and Elinor Goldschmied have kindly shared many valuable discussions with me for which I thank them.

Photographs have generously been given by Ted Remington, previously Assistant Head of Richard Cloudsley School, London EC1, who patiently took most of them, Christine White, formerly superintendent physiotherapist, and Miss Suckling, former head, and her staff were most helpful. Photographs for Figs 7.70, 7.137, 7.138, 8.3 and 10.1 were kindly given by The Cheyne Centre, Figs 7.173 and 7.176 by Professor K. Holt, Figs 7.95, 7.125–7.127, 7.129, 9.11 and 9.12 by Alison Wisbeach, The Wolfson Centre, Figs 5.2 and 5.5 by The Wolfson Centre Developmental Vision Clinic, Figs 7.67, 7.68, 7.209–7.212 by Ivan Hume and Figs 7.130

and 7.131 by The Foxdenton School, England. Photographs of examples of equipment were kindly given by James Leckey Designs, Jenx and Rifton Equipment.

My appreciation is given for the patient and critical reading of the manuscripts by my late husband Jack Halpern, Dr Peter Woolf, Dr Richard Lovell, Michelle Lee and various therapy colleagues. Typing by D. Wrathall, G. Smerdan, J. Deunette and M. Griffiths is gratefully acknowledged. The children and their parents who cooperated so amazingly with the long sessions of photography as well as all the children and parents I have been privileged to work with in the past and present have my heartfelt thanks.

My publishers have been particularly kind, helpful and sensitive and I thank Per Saugman, Peter Saugman and Staff of Blackwell Science.

A special thanks to my son David Halpern who as a boy showed much patience, understanding and skill in supplying numerous cups of coffee and now a great help in advice on editing and discussing my manuscripts.

Professor B. Neville has honoured me and encouraged me by writing the Foreword, for which I am most grateful.

Chapter 1
Principles of Treatment

The clinical picture in cerebral palsy

This chapter does not present the *medical aspects* in isolation, but outlines the clinical picture in such a way as to make it immediately relevant to the formulation of principles of treatment.

Cerebral palsy is the commonly used name for a *group* of conditions characterized by motor dysfunction due to non-progressive brain damage early in life. One could regard the cerebral palsies as part of a continuum of dysfunction which at one end merges into the field of severe or profound learning disabilities and at the other end into that of 'minimal brain dysfunction'. It is at this latter end that we find the clumsy children who are intelligent but have specific learning problems.

The motor dysfunction

In the past there was a tendency to look upon the various motor disorders only as problems of stiff or weak muscles or deformed joints. For whilst it is true that in particular cases the mechanical problems posed by these abnormalities have to be treated with orthopaedic and therapy procedures, this is but a small part of treatment as a whole. Many, if not all of the muscle and joint pictures encountered in the cerebral palsies arise from a lack of coordinating influences from the brain. In other words the neurological mechanisms of posture, balance and movement are disorganized. Therefore the muscles which are activated for controlling posture, balance and movement, become uncoordinated, stiff or weak. The therapist thus aims treatment primarily at the neurological mechanisms in the central nervous system which activate and control the muscles, within motor functions.

Principles of treatment of a number of therapists in the field largely centre on the spasticity, rigidity, athetosis or ataxia seen in children with the cerebral palsies. However, for therapy, it is far more important to concentrate on the overall functional loss which these and other physical problems create for these children.

Unfortunately, not all the neurological mechanisms which account for both normal and abnormal motor function of posture, balance and movement are fully understood as yet. Not surprisingly, different treatment systems offer different explanations and these are not always in agreement with research in the neurosciences. This book offers an approach to the postural mechanisms and movement which leads to a synthesis of many systems of treatment which have hitherto been widely regarded as being mutually exclusive. As a child does not move 'by neurophysiology alone' various ideas on learning motor control have been integrated into the general framework presented in this book. Chapter 3 will give principles of treatment, and Chapters 4 and 5 extend these principles to integrate the learning processes which may be involved.

Associated handicaps

Brain damage in cerebral palsy may also be responsible for special sense defects of vision and hearing, abnormalities of speech and language and aberrations of perception. Perceptual defects or *agnosias* are difficulties in recognizing objects or symbols, even though sensation as such is not impaired, and the patient can prove by other means to know or have known what the object or symbol is. There may also be *apraxias*, some of which are also called visuomotor defects. This means that the child is unable to perform certain movements even though there is no paralysis, because the patterns or *engrams* have been lost or have not developed. Apraxia can involve movements of the limbs, face, eyes, tongue or be specifically restricted to such acts as writing, drawing, and construction or even dressing. In other words there seems to be a problem in 'motor planning' in those children who are apraxic. Cerebral palsied children may also have various behavioural problems such as distractibility and hyperkinesis which are based on the organic brain damage. All these defects result in various learning problems and difficulties in communication. In addition there may also be various epilepsies or intellectual impairment (Foley 1977b; Hall 1984).

Not every child has some or all of these associated handicaps. Even if the handicap were only physical, the resulting paucity of movement would prevent the child from fully exploring the environment. He is therefore limited in the acquisition of sensations and perceptions of everyday things. A child may then *appear* to have defects of perception, but these may not be organic but caused by lack of experience. The same lack of everyday experiences retards the development of language and affects the child's speech. His general understanding may suffer so that he appears to be mentally retarded. This can go so far that normal intelligence has been camouflaged by severe physical handicap. Furthermore the lack of movement can affect the general behaviour of the child. Thus some abnormal behaviour may be due to the lack of satisfying emotional and social experiences for which movement is necessary. It is therefore important for any therapist to recognize that motor function cannot be isolated from other functions and that she is treating a child who is not solely physically but multiply handicapped.

Because of the multiple disabilities and lack of related learning experiences which interfere with a child's development, a physiotherapist or occupational therapist needs to be part of a team. The teamwork varies in different places such as community centres, child development centres, units in hospitals or within educational settings.

A team may consist of medical consultants in paediatrics, neurology, ophthalmology, orthopaedics, audiology and psychiatry with psychologists, physiotherapists, occupational therapists, speech therapists, teachers, nurses and social workers. Excellent progress has nevertheless been made by children with a much smaller and well integrated team including their parents and other family members, provided the whole child is considered.

The principle of teamwork varies from multidisciplinary, interdisciplinary and transdisciplinary approaches and is discussed in Chapters 4, 5, 8, and 10. Effective teamwork does not consist of separate assessments and isolated specialized treatments of specific disabilities by each team member as if they equal the 'whole' child. Although specialized work is important, attention must be given to the interplay that exists between all functional areas of a child. Assets in one function may be used to develop another different and inadequate ability. For example, speech may reinforce movement, motor activities stimulate speech, words and movement assist the training of perception and perceptuo-motor programmes develop understanding and language. The work of Stroh & Robinson (1986, 1991) is an example of functional learning which integrates motor, perceptual and emotional needs in the development of understanding and language. Interplay between apparently different developmental aspects is outlined in a book for parents and carers (Levitt 1994).

Aetiology

There are many causes of the brain damage, including abnormal development of the brain, anoxia, intracranial bleeding, excessive neonatal jaundice, trauma and infections. These have been extensively discussed in the medical literature (Crothers & Paine 1959; Bax 1964; Mitchell 1977; Hagberg *et al.* 1984; Stanley & Alberman 1984; Gordon & McKinlay, 1986). The therapist is, however, rarely guided by the aetiology in her treatment planning. In some cases the cause is not certain and in many cases knowing the cause does not necessarily indicate a specific diagnosis or specific treatment. Nevertheless, the therapist should acquaint herself with the history of the case. Many of these children have been affected from infancy and have been difficult to feed and handle. This may easily have influenced the parent–child relationships. Furthermore the history may sometimes give an indication of the prognosis, e.g. with marked microcephaly the prognosis would be poor.

Clinical picture and development

It is important to recognize that the causes of cerebral palsy take place in the prenatal, perinatal, and postnatal periods. In all cases, it is an immature nervous system which suffers the insult and the nervous system afterwards continues to develop in the presence of the damage. The therapist must therefore not think of herself as treating an upper motor neurone lesion in a 'little adult' nor can she regard the problem solely as one of retardation in development. What the therapist faces is a complex situation of pathological symptoms within the context of a developing child (Crothers & Paine 1959; Twitchell 1961, 1963, 1965; Peiper 1963; McGraw 1966; Denhoff 1967; Griffiths 1967; Sheridan 1973a, 1975; Egan *et al.* 1974; Holt 1975; Van Blankenstein *et al.* 1975; Illingworth 1975, 1980; Drillien & Drummond 1977, 1983). There are three main aspects to the clinical picture:

(1) Retardation in the development of new skills expected at the child's chronological age.
(2) Persistence of infantile behaviour in all functions, including infantile reflex reactions.
(3) Performance of various functions in patterns never seen in normal babies and children. This is because of the pathological symptoms of upper motor neurone lesions such as hypertonus, hypotonus, involuntary movements and biomechanical difficulties confronting children with cerebral palsy.

In order to recognize abnormal motor and general behaviour, the therapist should know what a normal child does and how he does it at the various stages of his development. Information on each handicapped child's developmental levels should be sought from the consultants and other members of the cerebral palsy team. Reference will have to be made to the extensive literature on the field of child development.

Although normal child development is the basis on which the abnormal development is appreciated, it does not follow that assessment and treatment should rely upon a strict adherence to normal developmental schedules. Even 'normal' children show many variations from the 'normal' developmental sequences and patterns of development which have been derived from the *average* child. The cerebral palsied child will show additional variations due to neurological and mechanical difficulties. If one considers, say, the normal developmental scales of gross motor development, the cerebral palsied child has frequently achieved abilities at one level of development, omitted abilities at another level and only partially achieved motor abilities at still other levels. There is thus a scatter of abilities.

If the gross motor development is generally considered to be around a given age, the development of hand function, speech and language, social and emotional and intellectual levels may all be at different ages. None of these ages may necessarily coincide with the child's chronological age.

Therefore the developmental schedules in normal child development should only be used as *guidelines* in treatment and adaptation should be made for each child's handicaps and individuality (Chapter 7).

More attention is usually given to motor development rather than other avenues of development, as it is the motor handicap which characterizes cerebral palsy. Here again, the therapist should remember that abnormal motor behaviour may interfere with other functions. Each area of development – such as gross motor, manipulation, speech and language, perception, social and emotional and mental – interacts as well as each having its own pattern or avenue of development. Therefore a total habilitation programme is necessary and should be planned to deal with the total development of the child.

Whilst aiming at the maximum function possible, the therapists concerned must take account of the *damaged* nervous system and adjust their expectations of achievements by the child which involve:

(1) Late acquisition of motor skills and slow rate of progress from one stage to the next.
(2) A smaller variety of skills than in the normal child.
(3) Variations in normal sequences of skills.
(4) Abnormal and unusual patterns of some of the skills.

Furthermore, the potential for function is dependent not only on the disabilities present, but also on the emotional and social adjustment of the child, his personality and 'drive' as well as his capacity to learn.

Change in clinical picture

As the lesion is in a developing nervous system the clinical picture is clearly not a static set of signs and symptoms for treatment. But whilst the lesion itself is non-progressive its manifestations change as the nervous system matures. As more is demanded of the nervous system the degree of the handicap appears to be greater. For example, a 3-year-old is expected to do more than a baby, and therefore his failures are greater for the same lesion.

In addition, the pathological symptoms may develop with the years. Spasticity may increase, involuntary movements may only appear at the age of two or three years, and ataxia may only be diagnosed when the child walks or when grasp is expected to become more accurate. Diagnoses may change as the baby develops to childhood, and especially as the child becomes more active. Later, especially in adolescence, growth and increase in weight contribute to apparent deterioration as the child matures.

Treatment minimizes the aggravation of symptoms. The earlier treatment is started the more opportunity is given for whatever potential there may be for developing any normal abilities and for decreasing the abnormal movement patterns and postural difficulties (Kong 1987; de Groot 1993). A baby or young child may make efforts to move using compensatory or adaptive patterns which can be 'good enough' but block the development of more efficient patterns or result in 'learned disuse' of a body part.

The value of early developmental intervention is to provide an increase in a baby's everyday experiences and interaction with his mother. The sooner a baby can be helped to move, the sooner he can explore, the sooner he can communicate the information he gains through such exploration. The therapist is in fact contributing to his learning and understanding as well as enabling him to bond with his mother.

Although the clinical picture is known to change with the years it is not yet possible to predict the natural history of the condition in each particular child. Infants and babies with marked early neurological signs may later prove to be only mildly affected, or even normal (Ellenberg & Nelson 1981; Nelson & Ellenberg 1982). On the other hand, apparently mildly affected ones may become progressively worse with the years. It is therefore difficult to prove the value of every early treatment. Nevertheless until we know which babies are going to 'come right' on their own, it is better to let them have the benefit of treatment so that any potentials for improvement are not lost. Despite the controversy as to the value of early treatment, there is clearly no doubt about its importance to the parents, who receive a great deal of practical advice and support from the therapists Among others, Goodman *et al.* (1991) found that if their research could not firmly state that neonatal physiotherapy was responsible for babies' motor developmental progress, all mothers confirmed their great appreciation for the support and practical ideas from their physiotherapists. Olow (1986) emphasizes that early intervention reduces the frustration of early rearing of children with disabilities. Whilst medical practitioners are watching the development of the child in order to make a reliable diagnosis, the parents have to live with that child throughout each day of those months and years.

Classification

Numerous classifications and subclassifications have been proposed by different authorities, but none of these diagnostic labels suffice to formulate adequate treatment plans. The therapist must also have a detailed assessment based primarily on motor functions, in order to work out a treatment programme.

CLASSIFICATIONS OF TOPOGRAPHY AND TYPES OF CEREBRAL PALSY

The topographical classifications frequently used are as follows:

Quadriplegia: Involvement of four limbs. Double hemiplegia is also used meaning that the arms are more affected than the legs and that there may be a congenital suprabulbar palsy.

Diplegia: Involvement of four limbs with the legs more affected than the arms.

Paraplegia: Involvement of both legs.

Triplegia: Involvement of three limbs.

Hemiplegia: One side of the body is affected.

Monoplegia: One limb is affected.

These topographical classifications are imprecise in that the other limbs may be slightly involved as well. The therapist should always consider whether or not she needs to include the 'uninvolved' limbs in her treatment. The hands of a paraplegic, for example, may need training in finer coordination or perhaps the other side of a hemiplegic may require treatment. The quadriplegics are often asymmetrical, with some of the limbs more obviously affected than the others. Triplegias and hemiplegias may really be quadriplegias. A pure monoplegia is almost non-existent.

The types of involvement are spasticity, rigidity, athetosis or hypotonicity. This latter called *atonic* cerebral palsy rarely remains hypotonic. These floppy babies usually become spastic, athetoid or ataxic. Athetoids and ataxics are mostly quadriplegic, but there is occasionally a hemiathetoid.

The classifications into types of cerebral palsy vary in different clinics but generally the main types are the *spastic*, the *athetoid* and the *ataxic*. Once again these classifications are not clear-cut and the therapist may have to treat symptoms of one type of cerebral palsy in another type. The predominant symptoms will contribute to the diagnostic type referred for treatment.

Spastic cerebral palsy

Main motor characteristics are:

Hypertonus of the *clasp-knife* variety. If the spastic muscles are stretched at a particular speed they respond in an exaggerated fashion. They contract, blocking the movement. This hyperactive stretch reflex may occur at the beginning, middle or near the end of the range of movement. There are increased tendon jerks, occasional clonus and other signs of upper motor neurone lesions.

Abnormal postures (see Figs 1.1–1.3) These are usually associated with the antigravity muscles which are extensors in the leg and the flexors

Fig. 1.1   Child with spastic
quadriplegia. Head preference
to right, shoulders protracted,
semi-abduction, elbows flexed-
pronated, wrists and fingers
flexed, thumb adducted. Hips and
knees flexed, tendency to internal
rotation-adduction with feet in
equino-varus, toes flexed.

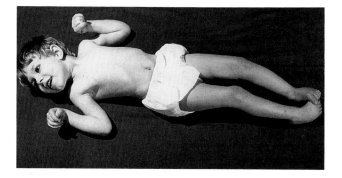

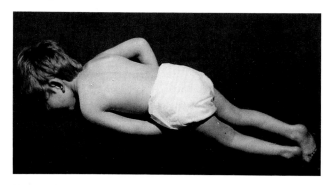

Fig. 1.2   Same child with
quadriplegia with postural
changes in prone. Asymmetry of
arms caught under body. Hips and
kness flexed, feet in equino-varus.
Head preference is now to left.

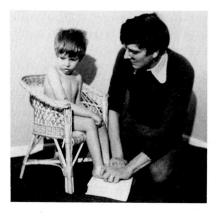

Fig. 1.3   Same child being taught
to sit by his father. Head
preference to right, shoulders
protracted, elbows flexed-
pronated, hands flexed, knees and
feet held symmetrical with hips.
Symmetrical trunk.

in the arm. The therapist will find *many* variations on this especially
when the child reaches different levels of development (Bobath & Bobath
1972). Common abnormal postures in supine, prone, sitting, standing,
walking and in hand function are described in Chapters 7 and 9.

The abnormal postures are held by tight spastic muscle groups whose
antagonists are weak, or apparently weak in that they cannot overcome
the tight pull of the spastic muscles and so correct the abnormal postures.

There are various other causes of abnormal postures which are discussed in Chapter 9. Abnormal postures appear as unfixed deformities which may become fixed deformities or contractures.

Changes in hypertonus and postures may occur with excitement, fear or anxiety which increases muscle tension. Shifts in hypertonus occur in the same affected parts of the body or from one part of the body to another in, say, stimulation of abnormal reactions such as 'associated reactions' or remnants of tonic reflex activity. Changes in hypertonus are seen with changes of position in some children. Position of the head and neck may affect the distribution of hypertonus. The latter are due to abnormal reflexes which may sometimes be found in these children. Sudden movements, rather than slow movements, increase hypertonus.

Hypertonus may be either spasticity or rigidity. The overlap between the two is almost impossible to differentiate. Rigidity is recognized by a *plastic* or continuous resistance to passive stretch throughout the full range of motion. This *lead pipe* rigidity differs from spasticity as spasticity offers resistance at a point or small part of the passive range of motion. For treatment planning the type of hypertonus is rarely important and techniques for motor development and prevention of deformity are the same.

Voluntary movement Spasticity does not mean paralysis. Voluntary motion is present and may be laboured. There may be weakness in the initiation of motion or during movement at different parts of its range. If spasticity is decreased or removed by treatment or drugs, the spastic muscles may be found to be strong, or may be weak. Once spasticity is decreased the antagonists may also be stronger once they no longer have to overcome the resistance of tight spastic muscles. However, in time these antagonists may have become weak with disuse.

The groups of muscles or *chains* of muscles used in the movement patterns are different from those used in normal children of the same age. Either the muscles which work in association with each other are stereotyped and are occasionally seen in the normal child, usually at an infantile level of movement, or the association of muscles is abnormal. For example, hip extension-adduction-internal rotation is used in creeping movements or in the push-off in walking but many other combinations must be used during the full execution of creeping and walking. This may be impossible in spastics who continue to use the same pattern at all times in the motor skill. Another example is shoulder flexion-adduction with some external rotation for feeding or combing one's hair in the normal arm pattern. In the case of the spastic, the arm pattern is usually flexion-adduction with *internal* rotation and *pronation* of the elbow. In taking a step in walking the normal pattern is flexion-adduction-external rotation at the hip, whereas the spastic pattern is frequently flexion-adduction-*internal* rotation of the hip. Other abnormal movement patterns occur as co-contraction of the agonist with the antagonist, instead of the normal relaxation of the antagonist. This blocks movement or makes it laboured. There are usually mass movements in that the child is unable to move an isolated joint. This absence of discrete movement is a characteristic feature of many spastics. Clearly there is not the smooth, co-ordinated, effortless and subconscious action of muscle patterns seen in normal motor skills.

General
(1)   Intelligence varies but may be more impaired than in children with athetoid cerebral palsy.
(2)   Perceptual problems, especially of spatial relationships, are more common in the spastic type of cerebral palsy.
(3)   Sensory loss occasionally occurs in the child with hemiplegia. There may be a visual field loss and lack of sensation in the hand. Growth of the hemiplegic limbs can be less than on the unaffected side.
(4)   Rib-cage abnormalities and poor respiration may exist.
(5)   Epilepsies are more common than in the other types of cerebral palsy.

Athetoid cerebral palsy

Main motor characteristics are:

Involuntary movements – athetosis   These are bizarre, purposeless movements which may be uncontrollable. The involuntary movements may be slow or fast; they may be writhing, jerky, tremor, swiping or rotary patterns or they may be unpatterned. They are present at rest in some children. The involuntary motion is increased by excitement, any form of insecurity, and the effort to make a voluntary movement or even to tackle a mental problem. Factors which decrease athetosis are fatigue, drowsiness, fever, prone lying or the child's attention being deeply held. Athetosis may be present in all parts of the body including the face and tongue. Athetosis may only appear in hands or feet or in proximal joints or in both distal and proximal joints.

Postural control   The involuntary movements or dystonic spasms may throw a child off balance. However, the well-known instability in athetoids is often directly connected with the postural mechanisms discussed in Chapter 2 (Foley 1983).

Voluntary movements   These are possible but there may be an initial delay before the movement is begun. The involuntary movement may partially or totally disrupt the willed movement making it uncoordinated. There is a lack of finer movements and weakness.

Hypertonia or hypotonia   Either may exist or there may be fluctuations of tone. Athetoids are sometimes called *tension and non-tension* types. There may be dystonia or twisting of the head, trunk or limbs. Sudden spasms of flexion or extension could occur. The hypertonia is a rigidity but occasionally spasticity may be present in the athetoid quadriplegias. Fluctuating tone sometimes occurs with fluctuations of mood or emotions.

The athetoid dance   Some athetoids are unable to maintain weight on their feet and continually withdraw their feet upwards, or upwards and outwards, in an athetoid dance. They may take weight on one foot whilst pawing or scraping the ground in a withdrawal motion with the other leg. This has been attributed to a conflict between grasp and withdrawal reflexes. This conflict of reflexes may also be seen in the hands (Twitchell 1961, 1963; Foley 1965).

Paralysis of gaze movements may occur so that athetoids may find it difficult to look upwards and sometimes also to close their eyes voluntarily.

Athetoids change with time   They may be floppy in babyhood and only exhibit the involuntary movements when they reach 2 or 3 years of age. Adult athetoids do not appear hypotonic but have muscle tension. Muscle tension also seems to be increased in an effort to control involuntary movements.

Subclassifications of athetoids vary from clinic to clinic. It is therefore particularly inaccurate to discuss the 'treatment of athetoids'. As mentioned above any classification changes with time. The therapist should treat the symptoms found rather than the subclassification.

General
(1) Intelligence is frequently good and may be very high. Intellectual impairment is occasionally present.
(2) Hearing loss of a specific high frequency type is associated with athetoids caused by kernicterus.
(3) 'Drive' and outgoing personalities are often observed among athetoids. Emotional lability is more frequent than in other cerebral palsies.
(4) Articulatory speech difficulties and breathing problems may be present.

Ataxic cerebral palsy

Main motor characteristics are:

Disturbances of balance   There is poor fixation of the head, trunk, shoulder and pelvic girdles. Some ataxics overcompensate for this instability by having excessive balance-saving reactions in the arms. Instability is also found in athetoids and spastics (see below).

Voluntary movements are present but clumsy or uncoordinated. The child overreaches or underreaches for an object and is said to have 'dysmetria'. This inaccurate limb movement in relation to its objective may also be accompanied by intention tremor. Poor fine hand movements occur.

Hypotonia is usual. Ataxia may be present in the hypertonic cases as well.

Nystagmus may exist.

General
(1) Intellectual impairment appears, especially in the presence of visual and perceptual problems.
(2) 'Clumsy' intelligent children are sometimes diagnosed as ataxic cerebral palsy.
(3) A 'pure' ataxic is rarely diagnosed.

Common features in all types of cerebral palsy

The classification into types of cerebral palsy tends to obscure the fact that there are important motor features which are common to all types. For instance, all cerebral palsied children are retarded in motor development. However the symptoms of the different types of cerebral palsy, such as hypertonus and the various involuntary movements, only play a part in this disturbance of development. Retarded or abnormal development of the postural-balance mechanisms or postural reflexes disturbs the motor development. Another common feature is the possible appearance of certain abnormal reflexes which have no predilection for a specific type of cerebral palsy.

Postural mechanisms (postural reflexes)

The inability to maintain posture and balance is most obvious in the athetoid children and children with ataxia, but is as much a cause of the physical handicap in the child with spasticity. Even if the spasticity were removed, the child would still be physically disabled (see Chapter 3 under the heading *Hypertonicity* in the section on the treatment of abnormal tone). The postural reflexes or postural mechanisms are neurological mechanisms which help to maintain posture and equilibrium and which are involved in locomotion. They have been described by various neurological workers. Purdon Martin (1967) has drawn on their work and, together with his own observations, presents a clear functional scheme which is described in Chapter 3 and related to development training and deformity in Chapters 4, 7, 8 and 9.

The postural reactions are an intrinsic part of motor skills. When they are absent or abnormal they lead to absent or abnormal motor skills. As the child acquires the different motor skills at various levels of development, he is in fact developing these postural mechanisms. Paediatric neurologists have studied ages in babies when certain postural reactions called *automatisms* appear with maturation. Terminology varies and Milani has grouped them into *righting reactions, parachute reactions* and *tilt reactions*. These need to be added to training of postural stability and counterpoising and all follow a general developmental sequence (see Table 6.2 and Fig. 6.2).

The postural mechanisms cannot be isolated from voluntary movements. Unfortunately some clinicians have overemphasized and isolated the problems of voluntary movement in the cerebral palsied child. The weakness and other abnormalities of voluntary movement have already been mentioned under the types of cerebral palsy. It is, however, important to understand that weakness of voluntary movement can also be bound up with the inadequacy of the postural mechanisms. When a child makes a voluntary movement, he has to maintain his balance as he does so. If equilibrium is inadequate the child may not be able to initiate a movement, or if he manages to carry out the movement on a background of unstable posture, that movement tends to be clumsy or uncoordinated. It is interesting to observe that during the development of hand function there is a period when the baby's hand skills are imprecise because his sitting balance has not been reliably established. It is therefore pointless for the therapist to train movements of arms or legs if the head and trunk are not being stabilized, with special methods.

Von Hofsten (1992), in discussing his many research studies on infants' visually directed reaching, had his infants fully supported. Their reaching became more successful as their postural control began at four months of age. Anticipatory postural adjustments of their trunks were observed at the normal age of nine months when these babies reached forwards. Hirschfeld (1992), Mulder (1991) and others quote many studies revealing that there is an anticipatory postural response before a voluntary movement is begun. This is a 'feed-forward' mechanism among others which are activated before a child voluntarily initiates movement. It is clear that there is close interaction between postural mechanisms and active limb movements (Belenkii *et al.* 1967; Marsden *et al.* 1981; Cordo & Nashner 1982).

One kind of weakness found in all cerebral palsied children is either of the muscles of head, trunk, shoulder and pelvic girdle or all of them. These are the muscles which are activated by the postural mechanisms. If these mechanisms are absent and the muscles cannot be activated, it is hardly surprising that they should be weak. One of the many reasons for floppy babies could be a lack of stimulation of the postural mechanisms. In cerebral palsied children floppiness of the head and trunk are also seen together with hypertonic limbs. This lack of development of head and trunk control is usually attributed to retardation of motor development. But this is in effect due to retarded development of the mechanisms of postural fixation of the head and trunk.

Abnormal reflexes (see Table 6.2)

Besides the desirable postural reactions, there are also reflexes which are undesirable. Many such pathological reflexes have been described in cerebral palsied children of all types. Diagnostic reflexes such as the tendon jerks, however, are of little relevance to treatment planning. Those reflexes which concern the therapist are some of the infantile or primitive reflexes. These are reflexes which are present in the normal newborn and which become integrated or disappear as the baby matures. In cerebral palsied children infantile reflexes are still present long after the ages when they should have become integrated within the nervous system. Whilst there are many infantile reflexes, those of most interest to the therapist are the Moro reflex, the palmar and plantar grasp reflexes, automatic stepping, excessive neck righting reflex, positive supporting, extensor thrust and feeding reflexes (Capute *et al.* 1978, 1984).

There are also the tonic reflexes, which are the tonic labyrinthine reflexes (TLR), the asymmetrical tonic neck reflex (ATNR) and the symmetrical tonic neck reflexes (STNR). Some neurologists group these tonic reflexes amongst the infantile reflexes whereas others argue that they are not present in the normal infant and are always pathological. These tonic reflexes are sometimes called *postural reflexes* but they are *abnormal* postural reflexes and should not be confused with the normal postural mechanisms as described by Rushworth (1961), Martin (1967), Foley (1977a), Roberts (1978) and others.

The principle of treatment which therapists should follow in relation to the complicated collection of reflexes is *not* to go 'reflex hunting'. Reflexes only concern the therapist when they interfere with motor function and speech. This does *not* always occur. The approach is to examine the function of the child first and only when abnormality has been detected, to then consider whether *one* of the reasons for this abnormality seems to be a pathological or primitive reflex.

Tonic reflexes are only seen in the most severely impaired children (Foley 1977), especially if obligatory. Table 6.2 and Fig. 6.2 of primitive and tonic reflex reactions are given so that a therapist recognizes any total or remnants of these reflex reactions or infantile (primitive) responses in individual children. These reactions may be stimulated by either peripheral or cortical activations. Some children with severe multiple disabilities activate some of these reflex responses in their efforts to communicate non-verbally. A therapist needs to include knowledge of how her peripheral stimulation and handling might cause undesirable reflex responses. However it is the therapist's work in building postural and movement control that does at the same time modify or overcome any undesirable reflex reactions.

Recent research calls into question the importance of primitive (infantile) reflexes. They are no longer considered a substrate for motor control and are not reliable predictors of future motor development. New ideas on theoretical bases of motor training disagree with using the 'hierarchical lists' of primitive and tonic reflexes followed by more mature reactions (Touwen 1976; Prechtl 1981; Cioni *et al.* 1989, 1992; Horak 1992). This increasing research on reflexes lends support to my view against reflex hunting expressed in this book since the First Edition in 1977.

Motor delay

Cerebral palsy consists of both motor delay and motor disorder. There are many other conditions which present similar problems of motor delay or of delay and disorder. All these conditions are also called the *developmental disabilities* (Pearson & Williams 1972).

They may be due to:

Intellectual impairment which is caused by various metabolic disorders, chromosome anomalies, leucodystrophies, microcephaly and other abnormalities of the skull and brain, endocrine disorders and the causes of brain damage given for the cerebral palsies. Down's syndrome also creates motor delay.

Deprivation of normal stimulation associated with social, economic and emotional problems, including maternal depression.

Malnutrition alone, but usually together with deprived environments. Once malnutrition is treated, lack of normal stimulation may still retard the child's development.

The presence of non-motor handicaps which may lead to motor delay, e.g. blindness, severe perceptual defects, apraxias, as well as intellectual disabilities mentioned above. Children with delay in any developmental area may have an associated delay in motor development (see the section on motor development and the visually handicapped child in Chapter 7).

Presence of motor handicaps other than the cerebral palsies For example spina bifida, the myopathies, myelopathies and various progressive neurological diseases and congenital deformities may obviously delay development, e.g. hand function has been delayed in children with spina bifida (Holt 1975) as well as gross motor development.

Principles of treatment and organization of treatment will be similar to that discussed in Chapters 3, 4, 5 and 8. *Specific problems* in the conditions above are considered in other publications (Shepherd 1980; Levitt 1984; Tecklin 1989; Campbell 1991; Eckersley 1993).

Principles of learning and therapy

Speech therapy and occupational therapy obviously overlap with education in drawing on principles of learning. Physiotherapy has 'grown up' predominantly within the fields of orthopaedics and neurophysiology. In recent years physiotherapists have recognized that it is no longer only a matter of working out what a child needs as treatment for medical problems but, also, how to enable a child to learn motor control.

Aims of physiotherapy, occupational therapy and speech therapy are:

(1) To develop forms of communication (gesture, speech, typing and alternative forms of communication with signs or electronic aids).
(2) To develop independence in the daily activities of eating, drinking, dressing, washing, toileting and general self-care.
(3) To develop abilities to play and achieve hobbies and recreational activities.
(4) To develop some form of locomotion and independent mobility which may include wheelchairs, playthings, electronic mobile buggies or driving motor vehicles.

All these aims need to be considered in terms of learning processes interacting with neurological and orthopaedic aspects. Therefore all therapists draw on the fields of education and psychology and gain much from close teamwork with teachers, psychologists, social workers and psychotherapists. The psychotherapists and social workers are important as learning is intimately involved with emotions. Many learning models do not give adequate attention to this fact.

Special equipment and adapted utensils, toys and other aids make learning of motor function easier. The child is more motivated to strive for independence and be rewarded by his own achievements.

Summary

Whilst it is difficult to summarize the principles of treatment concisely, the following points may be useful provided they are studied after reading Chapters 1 and 3.

(1) The child should be seen as being not only physically but multiply handicapped. In addition to motor dysfunction, associated disabilities may occur because of either brain damage, or lack of experiences due to inadequate movement, or both aspects combined.

(2) Treatment should be aimed at the neurological mechanisms of posture, balance and movement, supplemented by procedures for muscles and joints when necessary. This needs to be integrated into motor learning models.

(3) There should not be a rigid adherence to particular diagnostic classifications in treatment programmes, and aetiology may not influence the treatment in cerebral palsy.

(4) Emphasis should be given to training various postural mechanisms which are absent or abnormal in all types of cerebral palsy, or absent in any developmental motor delay.

(5) Treatment should also provide for features of the motor disorder such as hypertonicity, hypotonicity, involuntary movements, weakness, abnormal patterns of voluntary movements and abnormal reflexes *in the context of* total motor functions as well as in specific treatments for individual cases.

(6) The therapist should deal with abnormal reflexes only in those cases where they directly disrupt function.

(7) The therapist must deal with a complex situation of pathological symptoms within the context of a *developing* child in the cerebral palsies and other motor disorders.

(8) Developmental schedules of normal child development should only be used as guidelines and adaptations made to each child.

(9) Treatment should commence as early as possible.

(10) Treatment plans should be reviewed periodically to take account of changes in the clinical picture as the child grows older.

(11) Physiotherapists need to include learning principles in their work which also encompasses emotional issues.

Chapter 2
Outline of Treatment Approaches

There are many systems of treatment for cerebral palsy (Levitt 1962, 1976; Gillette 1969; Wolf 1969; Scrutton 1984). Although these therapeutic approaches were devised for the cerebral palsies, many of them are also used for treatment of children with other conditions of developmental delay and for adults with neurological defects. It is not the purpose of this chapter to describe each system in full detail and reference should be made to the literature and study observations of each system in practice. The author presents the essence of each system after many personal observations, discussions, practical work and reading of the work of the originators.

Muscle education and braces

W.M. Phelps, an orthopaedic surgeon in Baltimore, was one of the pioneers in the treatment of cerebral palsy who encouraged physio-therapists, occupational therapists and speech therapists to form them-selves into cerebral palsy habilitation teams (Egel 1948; Phelps 1949, 1952; Slominski 1984). The main points in his treatment approach were:

Specific diagnostic classification of each child as a basis for specific treatment methods. He diagnosed five types of cerebral palsy and many sub-classifications.

Fifteen modalities were described and specific combinations of these modalities were used for the specific type of cerebral palsy.
  The modalities (methods) were:

(1) Massage for hypotonic muscles, but contraindicated in spastics and athetoids.
(2) Passive motion through joint range for mobilizing joints and dem-onstrating to the child the movement required. Speed of movement is slower for spastics, increased for rigidity.
(3) Active assisted motion.
(4) Active motion.
(5) Resisted motion followed according to the child's capability.

  The above modalities were used for obtaining modalities 6, 8, 10 and 12.

(6)   Conditioned motion is recommended for babies, young children and mentally retarded children.

(7)   Confused motion or synergistic motion which involves resistance to a muscle group in order to contract an inactive muscle group in the same synergy. Mass movements such as the extensor thrust or the flexion withdrawal reflex are usually used. For example, using the hip-knee flexion dorsiflexion synergy, inactive dorsiflexors are stimulated by resistance given to hip flexors. Confused motion is further discussed in the sections on deformity.

(8)   Combined motion is training motion of more than one joint, such as a shoulder and elbow flexion using modalities 2, 3, 4, 5.

(9)   Relaxation techniques used are those of conscious 'letting go' of the body and its parts (Levitt 1962), and Jacobson's (1938) method of tensing and relaxing parts of the body. These methods are mainly used with athetoids. They attempt to lie still or relaxed or use contract-relax relaxation for grimacing and other involuntary motion.

(10)   Movement from relaxation is conscious control of movements once relaxation has been achieved. It is mainly used for children to control involuntary movements.

(11)   Rest – periods of rest are suggested for athetoids and spastics.

(12)   Reciprocation is training movement of one leg after the other in a bicycling pattern in lying, crawling, knee walking and stepping.

(13)   Balance – training of sitting balance and standing in braces.

(14)   Reach and grasp and release used for training of hand function.

(15)   Skills of daily living such as feeding, dressing, washing and toileting. Many aids were devised by the occupational therapists.

Braces or calipers   The appliances were designed and developed by Phelps. He prescribed special braces to correct deformity, to obtain the upright position and to control athetosis. The bracing is extensive and worn for many years. The children are taught to stand and step in long leg braces with pelvic bands and back supports, or sometimes spinal brace. As they progress, the back supports are removed, then the pelvic band and finally they wear below-knee irons. The full length brace has locking joints at hip and knee so that control can be taught with them locked or unlocked.

Muscle education   Spastics are given muscle education based on an analysis of whether muscles are spastic, weak, normal or *zero cerebral,* or atonic. Muscles antagonistic to spastic muscles are activated. This is to obtain muscle balance between spastic muscles and their weak antagonists. Athetoids are trained to control simple joint motion and do not have muscle education. Ataxics may be given strengthening exercises for weak muscle groups.

Others, including Deaver (1956), Rood (1956) and Tardieu (1973a,b), have developed ideas on bracing and muscle education. Deaver used braces for ambulation, eliminating brace elements as the child's control improved. He concentrated on self-care or activities of daily living, particularly the independent use of wheelchairs. Plum advocated strengthening spastic muscles as well as their antagonists. However, he exercised the spastic muscles in their outer ranges as the muscles are usually shortened, whereas the antagonists are exercised in their middle and inner ranges. Tardieu (1973b), in a 'factorial analysis' identifies the specific problem in the muscles which gives rise to abnormal movements or deformities. According to this careful analysis, treatment is given where indicated. Alcohol injections are used to diminish spasticity, muscle education, specific bracing and a preference for early orthopaedic surgery are recommended. Unlike most of the other orthopaedic approaches, Tardieu's includes neurodevelopmental studies. Tabary *et al.* (1972), Tardieu *et al.* (1982) and Dietz (1992) have shown specific changes in muscle length which warrant treatment in spasticity.

Progressive pattern movements

Temple Fay (1954a,b), a neurosurgeon in Philadelphia, recommended that the cerebral palsied be taught motion according to its development in evolution. He regarded ontogenetic development (in man) as a recapitulation of phylogenetic development (in the evolution of the species). In general, he suggested building up motion from reptilian squirming to amphibian creeping, through mammalian reciprocal motion 'on all fours' to the primate erect walking. As lower animals carried out these early movements of progression with a simple nervous system, they can similarly be carried out in the human in the absence of a normal cerebral cortex. The midbrain, pons and medulla could be involved in the stimulation of primitive patterns of movement and primitive reflexes which activate the handicapped parts of the body. Fay also described 'unlocking reflexes' which reduce hypertonus. Based on these ideas, he developed *progressive pattern movements* which consist of five stages:

Stage 1 Prone lying. Head and trunk rotation from side to side.

Stage 2 Homolateral stage. Prone lying, head turned to side. Arm on the face side in abduction-external-rotation, elbow semiflexed, hand open thumb out towards the mouth. Leg on face side in abduction, knee flexion opposite stomach, foot dorsiflexion. Arm on the occiput side is extended, internally rotated, hand open at the side of the child or on the lumbar area of his back. Leg on the occiput side is extended. Movement involves head turning from side to side with the face, arm and leg sweeping down to the extended position and the opposite occiput arm and leg flexing up to the position near the face as the head turns round.

Stage 3 Contralateral stage. Prone lying. Head turned to side, arm on the face side as in stage 2. The leg on the face side is, however, extended. The other leg on the side of the occiput is flexed. As the head turns this contralateral pattern changes from side to side.

Stage 4 On hands and knees. Reciprocal crawling and on hands and feet stepping in the *bear walk* or *elephant walk*.

Stage 5 Walking pattern. This is a *sailor's walk* called by Fay 'reciprocal progression on lower extremities synchronized with the contralateral swing of the arms and trunk'. A wide base is used and the child flexes one hip and knee into external rotation and then places his foot on the ground, still in external rotation. As the foot is being placed on the ground, the opposite arm and shoulder are rotating towards it. As weight is taken on the straight leg, the other leg flexes up.

The Doman-Delacato system (Doman & Doman 1960) which follows the basic tenets postulated by Fay, also recommends periods of inhalations of CO_2 from a breathing sack, restriction of fluid intake and development of cerebral hemispheric dominance. Cerebral dominance is attempted by principal use of dominant eye, hand, foot and arm and other methods. Children are also hung upside down and whirled around to stimulate the vestibular apparatus. They are also asked to hang and 'walk' their hands along a horizontal ladder as observed in apes.

The progressive pattern movements are first practised passively for 5 minute periods at least five times daily. One person turns the head, another person moves the arms and leg on one side, and another person the arm and leg on the other side. Locomotion beyond the stage of the child's patterning level is not permitted. A child who is not proficient in cross pattern creeping is prevented from walking. 'Neurological organization' is considered possible if each developmental level is established before going to the next level. This approach restricts itself to prone development and expects demanding daily regimes of treatment, amounting to 8–10 hours a day in many cases.

Synergistic movement patterns

Signe Brunnstrom (1970), a physical therapist, produces motion by provoking primitive movement patterns or synergistic movement patterns which are observed in foetal life or immediately after pyramidal tract damage. The main features of her work are as follows.

Reflex responses are used initially and later voluntary control of these reflex patterns is trained. Most of Brunnstrom's therapy has been on adult hemiplegics – in relation to the studies on the stages of recovery of flexion and extension limb synergies leading ultimately to isolated motion.

Control of head and trunk is attempted with stimulation of attitudinal reflexes such as tonic neck reflexes, tonic lumbar reflexes, and tonic labyrinthine reflexes. This is followed by stimulation of righting reflexes and later balance training.

Associated reactions are used as well as *hand reactions*, e.g. hyperextension of the thumb produces relaxation of the finger flexors. The training of a patient's voluntary control is developed later in the therapy programme.

Brunnstrom uses proprioceptive and other *sensory stimulation* in her training programmes for adult hemiplegics.

Proprioceptive neuromuscular facilitations

Herman Kabat, a neurophysiologist and psychiatrist in the USA, has discussed various neurophysiological mechanisms which could be used in therapeutic exercises. With Margaret Knott and Dorothy Voss, he developed a system of movement facilitation techniques and methods for the inhibition of hypertonus (Kabat *et al.*, 1959; Kabat, 1961; Knott & Voss, 1968; Voss, 1972). The main features of these methods are the use of:

Movement patterns (called mass movement patterns) based on patterns observed with functional activities such as feeding, walking, playing tennis, golf or football. These patterns are spiral (rotational) and diagonal with a synergy of muscle groups. The movement patterns consist of the following components:

(1) Flexion or extension.
(2) Abduction or adduction.
(3) Internal or external rotation.

Sensory (afferent) stimuli are skilfully applied to facilitate movement. Stimuli used are touch and pressure, traction and compression, stretch, the proprioceptive effect of muscles contracting against resistance and auditory and visual stimuli.

Resistance to motion is used to facilitate the action of the muscles which form the components of the movement patterns.

Special techniques

(1) *Irradiation* – this is the predictable overflow of action from one muscle group to another within a synergy or movement pattern or by *reinforcement* of action of one part of the body stimulating action in another part of the body.
(2) *Rhythmic* stabilizations which use stimuli alternating from the agonist to its antagonist in isometric muscle work.

(3) *Stimulation of reflexes* such as the mass flexion or extension.
(4) *Repeated contractions* of one pattern using any joint as a pivot.
(5) *Reversals* from one pattern to its antagonist and other reversals based on the physiological principle of successive induction.
(6) *Relaxation* techniques such as contract-relax and hold-relax. Ice treatments are used for relaxation of hypertonus.

There are various combinations of techniques.

Functional work or *mat work* involves the use of various methods mentioned above in training rolling, creeping, crawling, walking and various balance positions of sitting, kneeling and standing.

Neuromotor development

Eirene Collis (1947, 1953, 1956), a therapist and pioneer in cerebral palsy in Britain, stressed neuromotor development as a basis for assessment and treatment. Her main points were:

The mental capacity of the child would determine the results.

Early treatment was advocated.

Management – the word 'treatment' was considered misleading in that beside the physiotherapy session there should be 'management' of the child throughout the day. The feeding, dressing, toileting and other activities of the day should be planned.

Strict developmental sequence – the child was not permitted to use motor skills beyond his level of development. If the child was, say, learning to roll he was not allowed to crawl, or if crawling he was not allowed to walk. At all times the child was given a 'picture of normal movement' and, as posture and tone are interwoven, Collis placed the child in 'normal postures' in order to stimulate 'normal tone'. Once postural security was obtained, achievements were facilitated and developmental sequences were followed throughout this training.

The CP therapist Collis disliked the separation of treatment into physiotherapy, occupational therapy and speech therapy. She established the idea of the *cerebral palsy therapist*.

Neurodevelopmental treatment with reflex inhibition and facilitation

Karl Bobath, a neuropsychiatrist, and Berta Bobath, a physiotherapist, base assessment and treatment on the premise that the fundamental difficulty in cerebral palsy is lack of inhibition of reflex patterns of posture and movement (Bobath, B. 1965, 1971; Bobath, K. 1971, 1980; Bobath & Bobath 1972, 1975, 1984). The Bobaths associate these abnormal patterns with abnormal tone due to overaction of tonic reflex activity. These tonic reflexes, such as the tonic labyrinthine reflex, symmetrical tonic neck reflexes and asymmetrical tonic neck reflexes, have to be inhibited. They are not used in a reflex chart today, but are fundamental in treatment which 'counteracts the abnormal patterns of released postural reflex activity, and at the same time facilitates normal reactions by special techniques of handling' (Bobath 1984). Once the reflex patterns of abnormal tone are inhibited the child is said to have been prepared for movement. In addition, various primitive reflexes of infancy should also be inhibited. The main features of their work are:

Reflex inhibitory patterns specifically selected to inhibit abnormal tone associated with abnormal movement patterns and abnormal posture.

Sensory motor experience The reversal or 'break down' of these abnormalities gives the child the sensation of more normal tone and movements. This sensory experience is believed to 'feedback' and guide more normal motion. Sensory stimuli are also used for inhibition and facilitation and voluntary movement.

Facilitation techniques for mature postural reflexes.

Keypoints of control are used by the therapist to attempt to change the patterns of spasticity so that a child is prepared for movement and more mature postural reactions. The *keypoints* are usually head and neck, shoulder and pelvic girdles, but there is also work from distal keypoints. Abnormal tone is the cornerstone of this approach, which tries to 'normalize' it.

Developmental sequences were more strictly followed in the past, but are now modified according to each child.

All-day management should supplement treatment sessions. Parents and others are advised on daily management and trained to treat the children. Nancie Finnie (1974) has written a book for parents on this all-day handling of the child in the home.

Sensory stimulation for activation and inhibition

Margaret Rood, a physiotherapist and occupational therapist, bases her approach on many neurophysiological theories and experiments (Rood 1956, 1962; Stockmeyer 1967, 1972; Goff 1969, 1972). The main features of her approach are:

Afferent stimuli The various nerves and sensory receptors are described and classified into types, location, effect, response, distribution and indication. Techniques of stimulation, such as stroking, brushing (tactile); icing, heating (temperature); pressure, bone pounding, slow and quick muscle stretch, joint retraction and approximation, muscle contractions (proprioception) are used to activate, facilitate or inhibit motor response.

Muscles are classified according to various physiological data, including whether they are for 'light work muscle action' or 'heavy work muscle action'. The appropriate stimuli for their actions are suggested.

Reflexes other than the above are used in therapy, e.g. tonic labyrinthine reflexes, tonic neck, vestibular reflexes, withdrawal patterns.

Ontogenetic developmental sequence is outlined and strictly followed in the application of stimuli.

(1) Total flexion or withdrawal pattern (in spine).
(2) Roll over (flexion of arm and leg on the same side and roll over).
(3) Pivot prone (prone with hyperextension of head, trunk and legs).
(4) Co-contraction neck (prone head over edge for co-contraction of vertebral muscles).
(5) On elbows (prone and push backwards).
(6) All fours (static, weight shift and crawl).
(7) Standing upright (static, weight shifts).
(8) Walking (stance, push off, pick up, heel strike).

Vital functions A developmental sequence of respiration, sucking, swallowing, phonation, chewing and speech is followed. Techniques of brushing, icing, pressure are used.

Reflex creeping and other reflex reactions

Vaclav Vojta, a neurologist working in Czechoslovakia, now in Germany, developed his approach from the work of Temple Fay and Kabat (Vojta 1984, 1989; Von Aufschnaiter 1992). The main features are:

Reflex creeping The creeping patterns involving head, trunk and limbs are facilitated at various *trigger* points or *reflex zones*. The creeping is an active response to the appropriate triggering from the zones with sensory stimuli. The muscle work used in the normal creeping patterns or *creeping complex* have been carefully analysed. The therapist must be skilful in the facilitation of these normal patterns and not provoke pathological patterns. There are nine zones for triggering reflex locomotion.

Reflex rollings are also used with special methods of triggering.

Sensory stimulation Touch, pressure, stretch and muscle action against resistance are used in many of the triggering mechanisms or in facilitation of creeping.

Resistance is recommended for action of muscles. Various specific techniques are used to apply the resistance so that either a tonic or a phasic muscle action is provoked. The phasic action (through range) may be provoked on, say, a movement of a limb creeping up or downwards. The tonic action, or stabilizing action, is obtained if a phasic movement is prevented by full resistance given by the therapist. Therefore the static muscle action of stability occurs if resistance is applied so that it prevents any movement through range. *Rising reactions* are also provoked using resistance and all the methods above.

Conductive education

Andras Petö in Budapest, Hungary, originated *conductive education*. Since Professor Petö's death, the work has been continued by Dr M. Hari (Cotton 1965, 1968, 1970, 1974, 1975a,b; Hari *et al.* 1984, 1990; Beach 1988; Cottam & Sutton 1988). The main feature is the integration of therapy and education by having:

A conductor acting as mother, nurse, teacher and therapist. She is specially trained in the habilitation of motor disabled children in a four-year course. She may have one or two assistants.

The group of children, about fifteen to twenty, work together. Groups are fundamental in this training system.

An all-day programme A fixed time-table is planned to include getting out of bed in the morning, dressing, feeding, toileting, movement training, speech, reading, writing and other schoolwork.

The movements Sessions of movements take place mainly on and beside slatted plinths (table/beds) and with ladder-backed chairs. The movements are devised in such a way that they form the elements of a task or motor skill. The tasks are carefully analysed for each group of children. The tasks are the activities of daily living, motor skills including hand function, balance and locomotion. The purpose of each movement is explained to the children. The movements are repeated, not only in the movement sessions of, say, the *hand class* or *plinth work*, but also in various contexts throughout the day. The children are shown in practice how their 'exercises' contribute to daily activities.

Rhythmic intention The technique used for training the elements or movements is rhythmic intention. The conductor and the children state the intended motion: 'I touch my mouth with my hands'. This motion is then attempted together with their slow, rhythmic counts of one to five. Motion is also carried out to an operative word, such as 'up, up, up' repeated in a rhythm slow enough for the children's active movement ability. Speech and active motion reinforce each other.

Individual sessions may be used for some children to help them to participate more adequately in the work of the group.

Learning principles are basic to the programme. Conditioning techniques and group dynamics are among the mechanisms of training discussed. *Cortical* or conscious participation is stressed, as opposed to involuntary and unconscious reflex therapy. They feel reactions to handling cannot create active learning by a child.

Chapter 3
Synthesis of Treatment Systems

All the various treatment systems claim good results. It is difficult to decide which approach is superior whether on the basis of a scientific study or on theoretical grounds. Clinical experience of many therapists, as well as my own, has not confirmed the superiority of any one approach. The eclectic viewpoint has become increasingly accepted. In *Guidelines for Good Practice* (Dunn *et al.* 1990) there are statements such as recommendations to be 'selecting appropriately from the various approaches to management at each developmental stage'. In the USA, Umphred (1984) and Farber (1982) suggest integrated approaches quoting other colleagues who support this. Snell (1955), Decker (1962), Levitt (1962, 1969b, 1974), Gillette (1969), Hagbarth & Eklund (1969), Drummond (1977), McLellan (1984), Griffiths & Clegg (1988) and Dietz (1992) recognize elements of value in many different approaches and that common ground exists so that an eclectic approach is advisable.

A scientific study

This is fraught with many problems and to date no study to compare the value of different treatment systems has convincingly dealt with all the problems. Firstly, the results of treatment of the motor disability are influenced not only by the methods used, but also by the child's personality or 'drive', intelligence and home background as well as by the many possible associated handicaps of hearing, vision, perception or communication and by the presence of epilepsy. Matching children, apart from acquiring untreated controls, is difficult. One must also recognize that the enthusiasm, personality and skill of the therapist, rather than the particular system she is using, may have a strong effect on the results of treatment.

It is also difficult to compare systems of treatment by the records of the results achieved. The methods of assessment are often self-validating in terms of the theories of each system. Because the theories or concepts are controversial, such assessment of progress is not objective enough. In addition, therapists state the practical aims of particular methods in different ways. Achievement of any of these aims may be a 'good result' but may not make a great difference to the child's life. The superiority of different treatments cannot be assessed on the basis of these criteria. Any scientific study has to devise independent, valid and objective assessment techniques, as well as control the many variables and obtain untreated controls.

There are other problems. The results of a scientific study would have to be obtained over a long period of time. Crothers pointed out many years ago that one would really need a long-term follow-up to adulthood to establish the ultimate effects of treatment methods in childhood (Levitt 1962).

The research studies that have been carried out have been reviewed by Parette & Hourcade (1984) for the period 1952–82 and by Tirosh & Rabino (1989) for the period 1973–88. They all found in their reviews that the research designs were not rigorous enough and they discuss the problems that face researchers. Tirosh & Rabino suggest that a much larger number of subjects in a multicentre study should iron out the many variables and that more reliable data might be obtained. Meanwhile there has been an increase in single-subject studies to evaluate specific treatment procedures such as the use of below-knee plasters (inhibitory casts), ankle foot orthoses and similar procedures. Such studies offer a research design for physiotherapists, as discussed by Edwards *et al.* (1990), Riddoch & Lennon (1991) and Wilson (1987).

Specific treatment systems have been critically studied. The Doman-Delacato system was found unproven in results by Sparrow & Zigler (1978) and by Cummins (1988). Jones (1975), Bleck (1987) and Forssberg & Hirschfeld (1992) are critical of Vojta's approach. Vojta's list of postural reflexes is not accepted by Norén & Franzén (1982) as a reliable measure. The results of Vojta's early therapy as well as any other very early intervention cannot show that it was the intervention that obtained results and not the fact that many babies 'at risk' might have become normal anyway. Nelson & Ellenberg (1982) and Touwen (1987) point out how unreliable early diagnoses can be. Nelson & Ellenberg found in their large sample of babies suspected of cerebral palsy that there was a high rate of these babies becoming normal. Using proprioceptive neuromuscular techniques, Carlsen (1975) showed an improvement in a small sample of 12 children with cerebral palsy. Studies of conductive education in Britain (Bairstow *et al.* 1991, 1993) discuss the careful selection of children for this approach and a report in 1993 found that in a selected group, no difference was found between conductive education and the group in Manchester on a neurophysiological and developmental approach. Palmer *et al.* (1988) revealed that in the USA, neurodevelopmental treatment (NDT) was not as effective as a developmental stimulation programme for the whole child including motor development. The measure was the age of walking, but the quality of the walking patterns was not given clear attention. Bower & McLellan (1992), using an eclectic approach have shown the value of intensive therapy using an inter rater, intra rater reliable measure devised by Russell *et al.* (1989). The therapy was *eclectic*.

Theoretical grounds

Theoretical grounds for the different approaches depend on an understanding of brain function. This is highly controversial and cannot yet form a basis for the selection of the best treatment system. Every therapist wishes to understand 'why we do what we do' and, unfortunately, may accept a system because it offers a ready explanation. However, there is no all-encompassing theory that fully explains all the abnormal motor behaviour presented by the children, or the effects of various treatment procedures. Every system offers unproven neurophysiological and psychological hypotheses as well as reference to physiological experiments. Neuropsychology has rarely been used as a basis for treatment. Often normal physiology and normal child psychology are presumed to pertain to abnormal children. Is this necessarily so? And are the existing neurophysiological techniques subtle enough to bring about all the changes in the damaged nervous system that the theories claim?

Although the therapist should continue to ask herself why she is using a particular method, this enquiry should be focused on the observation of the behaviour of abnormal children and any changes in behaviour after treatment procedures. The reason for using a technique should not rest on theoretical hypotheses of brain function at this stage of our knowledge. We have to learn to live with that doubt.

Clinical experience

This has shown that choice of methods for an individual child depends on age, sex, personality and level of motor development. Developmental levels in other areas such as vision, hearing, communication, understanding and perception influence selection of techniques. Consideration has also to be given to facilities for treatment, the training of existing therapists, and the part played by the parents and the community, as to which methods are practical. If the therapist wishes to help as many children as possible, she must increase her repertoire of methods and not confine herself to the methods she has obtained in one system (Levitt 1962, 1969a,b, 1970b, 1974). Some of these methods cannot be learnt without long instruction in a special course on the system in which these methods occur. However, there are methods in every system which do not require the full specialized course in order to learn them. Someone who is trained in any system can select techniques from that system and teach them to a qualified physiotherapist. But, unfortunately, this does not happen as someone following a system often cannot divorce her techniques from the total system.

In the synthesis of treatment systems, I have offered principles of treatment which make it possible to select techniques from different systems according to the individual behaviour of the child. The techniques can be carried out by a qualified physiotherapist, although it is always preferable that she be supervised by senior colleagues and attend a course with an eclectic approach. Those directing these courses must themselves have studied many different systems and know what to select from them according to the aptitudes of the students.

The eclectic viewpoint in therapy

As it is difficult to confine oneself to any particular system and as each has made valuable contributions, an eclectic approach is recommended. In developing the eclectic approach, it has been necessary to try to understand the rationale underlying the methods in various systems of treatment.

At first, the systems appear different and even contradictory to one another. However, this is not really the case. Although there are differences, there is also common ground. The following discoveries emerged in my comparative study of the theory and practice of various treatment approaches:

(1) Different rationale are given by different systems for the same or similar methods. The common ground is the method, but the reasons offered differ.

(2) In some instances, the rationale are not really different, but only couched in different terminologies. The common ground is both the method and the reason for it.

(3) In other instances, the rationale are the same, only couched in different terminologies, but the methods suggested differ from system to system. The common ground is the rationale but methods differ.

(4) There are still differences in methods and rationale.

(5) Although methods may differ they are sometimes given the same name.

I have attempted to analyse and clarify this complicated field in order to bring together isolated but valuable pockets of knowledge. During these studies, it has also been difficult to know which methods and ideas in any particular system are the ones which are responsible for the results achieved. In any system there are methods and ideas which are superfluous. It is not correct that 'everything in a system depends on everything else'.

Methods and ideas have been selected rather more according to the problems of the children than according to the theories underlying the methods. In this way a synthesis of treatment can be made. This has now developed further and study continues in drawing on different models of motor learning to synthesize with therapy.

Synthesis of treatment systems

Despite different terminologies and methods the following aspects are fundamental to the various systems of treatment.

(1) The postural mechanisms.
(2) Voluntary motion.
(3) Perceptual motor function.

The postural mechanisms

Martin (1965, 1967) has studied and described the various postural mechanisms in a clear and practical way. I have found his particular presentation useful in clarifying the terminologies and methods in different approaches. His classification can also be used by the therapist in drawing on the various treatment approaches. In this book, it has been slightly modified and related to the problems of cerebral palsied children and other children who have motor delay.

The postural mechanisms are given and illustrated in the practical chapters. In outline they consist of:

The antigravity mechanism or the mechanism which helps to support the weight of the body against gravity.

This is also known as the *supporting reaction* in infants, *leg straightening reflex* or *positive statzreaktion*.

The postural fixation (stabilization) of parts of the body, i.e. head on trunk, trunk on pelvis and fixation of the shoulder girdles and pelvic girdles and the lower jaw, pharynx and tongue. Postural fixation of the body as a whole.

Terminologies also used for this are *stability, heavy work, tonic activity*.

Counterpoising mechanisms are closely associated with postural fixation. They are adjustments of the trunk and other parts of the body so that a movement can be made whilst the person maintains posture or equilibrium. Movements of the limbs or head provoke these adjustments of equilibrium.

Terminologies also used are *balance during motion, weight shifts, sway* and various *balance exercises* and *movement superimposed on co-contraction*.

Righting or rising reactions make it possible for the person to rise from lying to standing, or sitting to standing or many other changes of position. Rising into position as well as returning to the original position are both part of these reactions. Other terminologies used are *assumption of posture, moving into position* and *movement patterns*. The latter is confusing as there are also movement patterns which are voluntary movements and different to these automatic changes of posture. *Righting* is also used meaning either *sway* or *tilt* reactions and is not the sense in which I use it.

Tilt reactions occur when a person is tilted well off the horizontal plane and he adjusts his trunk so that he preserves his balance.

Reactions to falling or saving from falling These are various reactions in the limbs which prevent the person from falling over, if the tilt reactions cannot preserve balance. These reactions do not, on their own, stop falling over completely. For example, the arms may be thrown out to save the person from falling forward, sideways, backwards and in more complicated patterns. If the person is falling over from the standing position he may stagger, hop or quickly place a foot out to stop the fall. In sitting, kneeling and other positions the legs also move in order to save the person from falling from these positions.

Another terminology for these reactions is *protective responses*. Particular arm saving reactions are also called *parachute reactions, saving and propping on the hands, protective extension, arm balance responses, precipitation reaction* or *head protective response.*

Equilibrium reactions or *balance reactions* are also terms used which mean a combination of tilt and the limb reactions. These terms are confusing as all the postural reactions above are involved with equilibrium or balance. Maintaining a posture is synonymous with maintaining balance. Also, lack of tilt reaction seems to augment limb saving reactions and vice versa. This is seen in ataxic and athetoid children.

Whatever the terminologies and different viewpoints, these postural reactions are stimulated or trained within all systems of therapy. However, particular systems have emphasized some, but not all of these neurological mechanisms. Therefore it is important to draw on all systems to make sure that none of the child's postural mechanisms are neglected. In addition, those systems that have given attention to all these problems have not necessarily suggested methods to cover the needs of all children and once again selection of methods is essential when children do not respond.

Besides the six main postural reactions above, there are also:

Locomotive reactions which serve to initiate stepping, continue stepping and stop stepping.

Ocular postural reflexes and control of facial musculature are also interwoven with the postural mechanisms.

These reactions can be stimulated within developmental training, using methods drawn from different systems of treatment. It is helpful to follow motor developmental levels, for as the child acquires the motor abilities in these sequences, he is acquiring these neurological mechanisms. However, the sequences may vary in normal and abnormal children. This is discussed below in the section on developmental training.

Voluntary motion

Voluntary motion which is purposeful, conscious, willed motion is sometimes confused with the active automatic movements which occur in the postural mechanisms such as rising or saving from falling. Although some of the automatic movement synergies are also seen in voluntary movement, stimulation of the automatic patterns only corrects abnormal postures and movements but does not contribute enough to the training of voluntary motion. Voluntary motion uses many different synergies and there may be a great variety of synergies in any one child for the same task. In time he chooses the most effective pattern. Voluntary motion is also bound up with postural mechanisms in that they help to create stable posture so that limbs can be accurately used. Arm function and hand movements themselves activate postural fixation and counterpoising of the trunk, and the shoulder girdle for coordination. The proximal-caudal rule in development is therefore inaccurate. Postural fixation and counterpoising of the head also helps eye–hand coordination. Vision affects postural control (see the section on motor development and the visually handicapped child, in Chapter 7, and the review by Sugden 1992).

Voluntary motion is, however, far more complex, in that it is involved with perceptual, praxic and cognitive function. Physiotherapists contribute neuromuscular techniques which need to include more than the stimulation of automatic arm and leg patterns of postural reactions. These patterns are drawn from many systems of treatment and are discusssed in particular reference to arm and hand function in Chapter 7. Additional advice must be obtained from other disciplines working on the learning of motor skills, i.e. psychology, special education and physical education.

Perceptual motor function

The therapy systems explored in this book touch on the role of the physiotherapist, occupational therapist and speech therapist's contributions to stimulation of all the senses, linking of sensations, sensory discrimination, developing body image, body scheme, spatial relationships and direction and other aspects which are related to perceptual motor function. The psychologist, occupational therapist, teacher and other specialists make specific structured contributions to these aspects. The neuromuscular techniques in the various therapy systems may be integrated with the perceptual motor training, usually part of occupational therapy (Morgenstern *et al.* 1966; Brereton & Sattler 1975; Ayres 1979; Fisher *et al.* 1991).

Treatment principles for a synthesis of therapy systems

The common ground between the different systems forms the principles of treatment. These common denominators will be discussed so that the therapist can understand where they exist and where differences are apparent or real.

General principles of treatment which are commonly accepted by various schools of thought are:

(1) Team work.
(2) Early treatment.
(3) Repetition of a motor activity, whether it is neuromuscular techniques in treatment sessions or in the motor activity during all-day management.
(4) Training of parent either for home treatments or practical management. Motivation of child and parent.

Specific principles of treatment   Common factors detected in the various systems of treatment are:

(1) Developmental training.
(2) Treatment of abnormal tone.
(3) Training of movement patterns.
(4) Use of afferent stimuli.
(5) Use of active movement.
(6) Facilitation, abnormal and normal 'overflow'.
(7) Prevention of deformity.

Developmental training

Most systems of treatment suggest following the normal motor developmental sequences of child development. It is, however, superficial to advise therapists, as is frequently done, 'to follow normal motor developmental sequences'. Viewpoints differ as to whether to strictly follow these sequences, or modify them. Viewpoints also differ as to whether to train a total motor function such as rolling, crawling, standing or walking (Denhoff & Robinault 1960; 'Mother treatment' in Gillette 1969) or whether to break each function down into elements for training (Rood 1962; Cotton 1975a; Bobath & Bobath 1975; Levitt 1986, 1991; Vojta 1989; Levitt & Goldschmied 1990). Most therapists prefer to train elements or *bricks* which build up the motor function as well as train the total function. However, views differ as to what these elements are. Some talk of different types of muscle tone, different reflexes, different muscle work and other ideas. In addition, *basic motor patterns* are recommended as the basic abilities which underlie many motor functions on the develop-

to 'throw the child off balance', but may not prevent the development of the postural reactions. The association of these athetoid symptoms and postural reactions is not clear yet. Severe athetoids have disrupting spasms or tone fluctuations and severe disability in function. Nevertheless in some children voluntary motion can be trained, despite disturbance by the involuntary movements. Improvement of postural mechanisms seems to *decrease* the disrupting effect and sometimes the degree of involuntary motion.

To summarize   The therapist should not collect techniques for abnormal tone *as such* but rather:

(1)   Emphasize training the motor functions composed of postural reactions and voluntary motion.
(2)   Enlarge the amount and variety of motor abilities.
(3)   Train the best pattern of performance so that deformity is prevented or decreased.
(4)   Concentrate on threatening and established deformities which may block function, e.g. spastic plantarflexors which contribute to toe standing and increase difficulty in sitting. A secure base is needed and provided by a pair of feet held flat on the ground.

The treatment of deformity involves many methods as well as orthopaedic surgery and the use of splintage, plasters and special equipment (see Chapter 9).

Training of movement patterns

Some therapy systems assess and treat individual muscle groups (Phelps 1952; Plum & Molhave 1956; Slominski 1984) and this muscle education is associated with orthopaedics (Sharrard 1971; Samilson 1975). Apparently contradictory views are held in the neurological approaches, which strongly recommend assessing and training movement patterns, and patterns of posture. There is no total contradiction for the following reasons:

(1)   Movement patterns are made up of muscle groups. In fact Tardieu (1973a,b) points out that *movement pattern* is a vague term as movement patterns may look the same, but be composed of different muscle actions in different children. Holt (1965, 1966) demonstrates with electromyography that the muscles acting in the same pattern of posture are different in different children. In orthopaedics, particular joints may be more deformed than others so that presumably some muscle groups are more troublesome than others *within* any abnormal patterns. It is therefore helpful to analyse the muscle work in abnormal patterns of movements and posture with

electromyography and clinical observation as for example in gait analyses (Leonard *et al.* 1988, 1991).

(2) Although individual muscle groups may be assessed *in isolation a* is usual in orthopaedic physiotherapy, there is no need to follo such assessments with isolated muscle education. Muscle educati can be obtained *in pattern* as well. At low levels of development f child cannot easily isolate his movements. More severely br damaged children and adults can only use mass movements synergies of muscle action and cannot respond to localized mu education.

(3) Besides the level of function of any particular child, there is also a. fact that training a muscle group, or relaxing a spastic muscle group, does not guarantee that the particular muscle group will work correctly within a function. Muscles are activated as prime movers, synergists or fixators when they contract, as well as being inhibited (relaxing, 'letting go') as antagonists, during motion. Muscles have to shorten and contract (concentric work or isotonic), keep the same length and contract (isometric work) or lengthen and contract (eccentric work) in different movements. These various muscle actions are best trained in the movement in which they will be used in motor function (see Task analysis in Chapter 4; The therapist's specialized assessment in Chapter 5 and the Summary, of specific deformities, in Chapter 9).

Movements are presented as various movement patterns by different treatment systems. Movement patterns are often considered separately from a motor function and are:

Movement patterns seen in the infant's spontaneous motility and in the infantile reflex reactions (Table 6.2) such as the Moro, the tonic neck, the withdrawal and crossed extension reactions and many others (Capute *et al.* 1984). There are also the spontaneous movements seen in normal infancy, which are now considered of special importance for study (Touwen 1976; Prechtl 1981; Cioni *et al.* 1992; de Groot 1993).

Movement patterns preferred by brain damaged patients which include normal primitive synergies such as the flexor synergy of hip flexion-knee flexion-dorsiflexion (the withdrawal reflex, mass flexion reflex, von Bechterew reflex or Strumpel's phenomena) or the extensor synergy of hip extension-knee extension-plantarflexion (extensor thrust), and crossed extensor reflex which is the flexor synergy in one leg with the extensor synergy in the other leg. There are also various abnormal patterns which are not primitive, in the sense that they may not be seen in normal infants, but which are only seen in neurological cases with damage to the central nervous system. These are being studied in ongoing research in pre-terms, full-terms and older babies. Examples already known are opisthotonus, severe asymmetries and dystonias in older children. (See Table 6.2.)

Mature patterns of movement seen in older children and adults. These patterns have more rotation and a variety of combinations of flexion and extension within any one synergy.

As the former two problems are indications of abnormality in children at six months of age and older, some therapists will not use these patterns in any children over six months. There are, however, children who are so immobile and severely handicapped that the primitive patterns are the only ones which are possible. The reflex creeping complex, reflex rolling, withdrawal reactions or automatic stepping may be used to provoke movement. Such movement is also selected to counteract persisting abnormal postures. A severe spastic may lie stiffly with his legs in extension-adduction-internal rotation. The legs will move into flexion-abduction-external rotation if reflex forward creeping is provoked. Fay (1954a,b) called the reflex flexion and other reflex motion *unlocking reflexes* as they unlocked a spastic position or pattern. Egel (1948), Snell (1955), Brunnstrom (1970) and Slominski (1984) are some workers who found they could only achieve action of an inactive muscle group if this muscle group could be activated within these primitive synergies. Lack of action in particular muscle groups contributes to deformity and therefore these synergies variously termed *mass reflexes, synkinetic motion, confused motion, primitive reflex patterns*, were used.

It is, however, desirable to attempt more mature patterns if they are possible. These are for example the patterns of Kabat's *mass movement patterns* seen in functional activities (Kabat 1959, 161; Knott & Voss 1968), and Bobath's mature patterns in the developing child (Bobath 1971; Bobath & Bobath 1975, 1984).

In the treatment of one child at one level of function, it would be contradictory to use methods for reflex movement patterns seen in brain damaged children or normal infants together with methods for mature synergies seen in normal young children or adults. The therapist uses only those techniques which relate to the level of development or capacity of any particular child's nervous system.

To summarize Considering the many different methods used for muscle education and movement pattern training, it is *generally* advisable to 'Stimulate movements initially through primitive mass patterns, reflexes (Fay, Kabat), confused motion (Phelps) or through synkinetic movements (Snell) for the severely impaired children. Whenever possible it is best to modify these primitive combinations of movements into more controlled and advanced patterns (Kabat, Bobath) and finally into selective or isolated movements (Phelps, among others)'. Hellebrandt summarises Coghill as saying 'that the earlier manifestations of movement are perfectly integrated total patterns within which partial patterns arise, acquiring various degrees of discreteness by a process of individuation' (Levitt 1962). The different patterns of movement in normal and abnormal motor development and the techniques of therapy for muscle work and movement pattern are discussed in the chapters on developmental training, and prevention and correction of deformity.

Recent work discussed in Chapters 4 and 5 emphasizes that although all these movement patterns do help to reduce muscle tightness, mobilize joints and obtain motion in an otherwise immobile child, these movement patterns need to be used in the context of activities which are of interest to a child to solve problems in his daily life. Facilitating automatic movement patterns or any movement patterns in isolation do not transfer into whole motor function. A child has to be enabled to learn how to do this.

Use of afferent stimuli: automatic and conscious motor activity

Most treatment systems use afferent stimuli of touch, temperature (cutaneous) or pressure, stretch, resisted motion, joint compression or retraction (proprioceptive stimuli) as well as visual and auditory stimuli. With various methods, therapists use their hands on the child to elicit muscle actions, reduction of spasticity and stimulate movement patterns. These motor activities are often reflex responses, i.e. on an automatic level. The child 'reacts to the stimuli' and feels a movement or posture he cannot achieve himself. In time this sensory-motor experience helps him acquire the motion or posture on his own. The action of the muscles within the response of automatic movement or muscle action is *active* as opposed to *passive* motion. What is not active is the child's initiation of the motion or the child's active concentration or participation in carrying out the patterns of movement and postures. His active efforts are considered to increase spasticity or abnormal patterns of function (Bobath & Bobath 1984; Vojta 1989). Rood is quoted as saying 'let us use our heads to do other things than run our muscles' (Goff 1969). It is emphasized that our muscle actions, movement synergies and postures are not carried out at a conscious level but on an involuntary, unconscious level. When we move and balance, we do not think of these actions.

It is important to recognize that movements and postures are involuntary *after* they have been achieved. In the process of training motor function as, say, in learning to drive a car, play tennis or ice skate, concentration on the movement and equilibrium is needed. Children should concentrate on, say, movements for rising from the floor, on maintaining balance, on putting their hands out to save themselves, to stop themselves from falling during training. For example, blind children have been taught to save themselves with verbal instructions to 'put out their arms' (observed by Zinkin 1976). Later this becomes automatic. Automatic reactions may be possible in some procedures and should also be provoked this way if it is possible.

The child should also have his conscious attention on the afferent stimuli used by the therapist, as they are often cues to direction or to parts of his body and convey what movement is required. In addition, the child can be asked to 'pull', 'push', 'stretch up', 'try to sit alone' and so on. Some children, especially younger and mentally low children, respond better to concentration on an incentive for a particular motion, 'touch this', 'catch this', and on the motivation of toys and play. Neurophysiological techniques to facilitate automatic motion and counteract abnormal motor activity have obviously to be interwoven with the child's conscious participation (see Chapters 4 and 5).

The Petö approach is particularly careful to use the child's *cortical* or conscious control of motion (Cotton 1970, 1974, 1975b). However, this approach does not carry out every aspect of motion consciously. The active efforts may focus on, say, voluntary arm motion whilst automatic head and trunk control occur. Conscious actions that are selected do not aggravate spasticity as these active motor activities are not too far ahead of the child, so that he is *pushed* to make abnormal efforts to achieve a movement. The afferent stimuli are contained in the auditory and visual stimuli in the instructions the children use. *Fixation* of a part of the child's body may involve manual contact with the child. However, little of the training of motion is based on afferent stimuli by the therapist handling the child.

To summarize   It is advisable to show the child how and where to move by the therapist's afferent stimuli for automatic movements and postures. However, as soon as possible and even in the same therapy session, check whether the child can carry out the motor activity on his own even though it will be partial or unreliable. He should then concentrate and practise the motor activity without being handled or touched by the therapist. The motor activity selected should be at his level of development so that he can achieve something on his own. The child gains more from any corrective motor activity that he does himself. If, however, the child is so severely disabled that there is no activity possible on his own, facilitation with afferent stimuli or handling may be the only way to begin motor activity. Taub (1980), Rothwell (1982), Gordon (1987) and others have drawn attention to research that shows that movements can be achieved without afferent input. However, Rosblad & von Hofsten (1992) demonstrated that sensory input is essential for fine coordination. There is a central motor programme in a child's central nervous system which can be used without afferent stimuli. Afferent stimuli are, however, needed to modify the child's actions and achieve accuracy of motor control. 'Hands on' sensory stimuli are therefore not always necessary.

Passive or active motion

Zuck *et al.* (1952) and others have shown that active movement obtained more progress than passive procedures of passive motion and bracing. Passive *patterning* of children or a *full range of passive motion* cannot contribute much, if anything, to training motion. They only keep the joints mobile, and help to prevent deformity.

Passive correction by splintage, plasters or orthopaedic surgery passively changes the child's positions so that he obtains a better proprioceptive experience or position from which to develop active motor function. Passive correction of, say, the child's feet in plasters makes his active correction of knees and hips and balance possible.

Passive motion may be used to show the child what motion is required, but afferent stimuli are more effective as the active response to these stimuli gives a better proprioceptive as well as visual-auditory demonstration of what is required. Active or active resisted motion provides better proprioceptive information than passive motion (Kabat *et al.* 1959; Kabat 1961; Held 1965).

The previous section on automatic and conscious movement should also be read to obtain the whole picture of the controversy of active and passive therapy. The chapter on learning motor function emphasizes the need for *active* motor function.

Facilitation, abnormal and normal overflow

Many systems of treatment have used the activation of one part of the body to facilitate action in another part of the body, e.g. arm elevation simultaneously activates head elevation and back extension, creeping techniques triggered at the legs facilitate activity in the whole child. Stimulation of one part of a synergic movement pattern activates the other muscle groups within the same synergy. These facilitation techniques involve normal *overflow* of activity from one area of the body to another. Feldenkrais (1980) has made an intensive study of such interactions in the whole normal body.

It is, however, possible to activate undesirable actions in other parts of the body, e.g. grasping may increase flexion in the elbows and shoulders in a child already round-shouldered and flexed, use of the arms may increase spastic abnormal postures in the legs and grasping with one hand may be associated with clenching of the other hand. There are other abnormal *associated reactions* observed by Bobath. Repetition of such abnormal overflow, as opposed to the normal overflow of facilitation techniques, may aggravate abnormal postures and increase deformities. Facilitation techniques, including afferent stimuli and the use of resisted motion, must be used in such a way that the rest of the body does not become abnormal (Levitt 1966, 1967, 1969c, 1970b).

In this context it is important to combine the ideas of Bobath with those of Knott in facilitating motion. Knott facilitates motion in one part of the body with afferent stimuli and resistance. The rest of the body must be *positioned* so that abnormal overflow does not occur. Vojta's techniques use resistance to creeping but, as the whole body is moving in a corrective pattern, positioning is unnecessary. Also much rotation within facilitation patterns in spastics prevents overflow of spasticity to other parts of the body.

To summarize Any patterns facilitated in one part of the body should be accompanied by careful observation of the whole child and not only of the part being activated. Normal or abnormal overflow of motor activity should be observed when using techniques in one part of the body to facilitate activity in other parts of the body. Physiotherapists can learn more about normal interactions of body parts in their own experience in 'Feldenkrais classes' (Feldenkrais 1980).

Prevention of deformity

Every system aims to prevent or correct deformity. There are many methods to counteract deformity as well as many viewpoints as to the genesis of deformity. Chapter 9 is devoted to this aspect.

Chapter 4
Learning Motor Function

Therapists point out that most learning processes are dependent on the ability to move. Therefore motor function is stimulated and developed with neurophysiological techniques drawing on one or more systems. Once the ability to move is achieved, this is then applied to learning self-care, classroom activities, play and hobbies, household chores and later work. It is important to consider that a child does not move by neurophysiology alone:

- A child with brain damage *learns* motor functions such as sitting, standing, changing postures, using hands and the various forms of locomotion.
- A child *learns how* to use equipment such as walking aids, wheelchairs and playthings.
- A child *learns to* use his motor functions to achieve self-care, play and interaction with people and objects in most daily tasks.

Studies and clinical experience now show that activation of muscles or motor patterns on their own can show an improvement, but this is a performance in a therapy session and is not necessarily learnt. The improved motor performance does not transfer into the actions of daily life (Goldkamp 1984; Gordon 1987; Mulder & Hulstijn 1988). In the next chapter I have been starting with motor patterns in the context of the daily lives of children and their parents based on the need to translate my technical knowledge into what has meaning for them (Levitt 1986, 1991, 1994). This is followed by specific practice of any motor patterns which are inefficient and by activation of motor actions which are dormant but necessary for any daily life activity. Any improvement in motor pattern is immediately used within the daily task at the same session.

Learning methods

Many experienced paediatric physiotherapists and occupational therapists do intuitively select training methods which suit an individual's learning style. This art and common sense of therapists can be supported by some of the knowledge and research presented by experts in the behavioural sciences. It is nevertheless of much value to learn from such experts so that a therapist comes to understand more deeply and analytically what she is already doing so that she can be more precise in the way that she works. These studies also offer theories for our work and new ideas are likely to be developed, (Carr *et al.* 1987; Mulder 1991; Forssberg & Hirschfeld 1992).

A behaviour

This is a term used by psychologists and teachers to convey any action of a child that can be observed. When behaviours are troublesome for therapists and parents in that a child refuses to cooperate, dislikes handling or having splints applied then these are discussed with team members. A clear description of what a child does, when he does it and people's responses to his behaviour is discussed so that a constructive approach can be worked out.

The behaviours which are more directly the concern of physiotherapists are motor acts. A description of what a child does with the criteria for success of a motor act is called *behavioural objective* for therapy (Presland 1982; Steel 1993). For example, 'Sitting on a potty for one minute independently without extending backward or falling to the right' (Bower & McLellan 1992). This gives the motor act, how it is done and for how long. We need to go further and state a carer's or a therapist's response to a child's motor function as is done with other behaviours. This will affect a child's learning of any motor function. A carer may face and talk to a child or look approvingly at his achievement or calmly ignore it when he does not succeed (see below).

The development of a child's attention

Cerebral palsies may create apathy, hyperactivity and fleeting attention in children. Besides the brain damage which causes these difficult behaviours, they may be due to some drugs, exhaustion and emotional stress of a child. His refusal to cooperate and concentrate also has a number of other explanations. Parents find their child's poor concentration and restlessness very demanding (French & Patterson 1992). They are enabled to understand that therapy depends on concentration by a child on a number of tasks at his level of development which will therefore improve not only the tasks but his attention span. Therapy needs concentration and is not necessarily only a set of automatic movement responses or specialized neuromuscular procedures during which a child 'receives treatment'.

Ideas to promote attention and learning

(1) The programme is at each child's stages of motor, sensory, perceptual and cognitive development.
(2) Use small steps within each stage so that achievement is possible. Successful achievement maintains attention.

(3) Impairments are known so that the influences of other disabilities are appreciated.

(4) Difficult and new motor tasks need to be interspersed with easier ones.

(5) Ensure that the therapy session does not have too many activities and that priorities are chosen.

(6) The time of day must be considered. A child may be better in the morning or some time after a meal or rest. Clearly, concentration of a child is not enhanced if he is taken away for therapy from his favourite lesson in school or from a special hobby or play activity.

(7) The length of a therapy session must relate to the child's attention span.

(8) Avoid distractions of too many people moving around, too much noise or non-stop television or radio during sessions.

(9) A child's attention is best appreciated in terms of his stage in the usual sequence of development of attention, so that too much is not expected of him. Infants normally attend to more of their internal activities and to stimulation very close to them. Around 6 to 12 months their attention can be focussed on stimuli of sight and sound further away from them. Fleeting attention in infants becomes longer in duration until they focus rigidly on one thing at a time. Later they will allow an adult to shift their attention and become more flexible in use of their attention (Cooper *et al.* 1978).

Learning a motor function

When a child focuses his attention on a motor task, he is more likely to learn it. The therapist clarifies for him where he needs to concentrate. In the first stage a child focuses his attention on the purpose for moving. This is his *intention* to move or the *action goal*. This may be a child's daily living activity of, say, eating, washing, dressing or interacting with his mother or other family member. It may be exploring an object or getting to a place where he wants to be.

Once focused on the goal, the child uses what are called *goal-directed movements* together with postural mechanisms. His attention is kept on the task as he learns which motor actions are used to achieve this goal. Therapists need to avoid *goal confusion* by their emphasis on the *best motor pattern* rather than maintaining a child's attention on the goal (Gentile 1987). Once some understanding of what to do is shown by a child, then his attention shifts more to how to do it. The action of movement and posture is therefore not separated from the purpose of that action.

A child's own goals and strategies

A learning model often involves an adult explaining what a child is going to do, showing him how to do it and keeping his attention on these aspects. However, if one precedes this approach with discoveries of what a child himself wants to achieve, he may not need to have explanations of what he is going to do. If a therapist also observes how he goes about trying to achieve his own goal *she* learns about his motivation and what he can already do using his choice of postural controls and movement patterns (see Fig. 4.1). These may be:

- An approximation of the whole task.
- An initiation of the task without completion.
- An unusual way of doing the task.

The therapist can then show that child how to develop or modify the task if his approximation of a task is at a *lower developmental stage* of performance, *uses symptoms* of his type of cerebral palsy, *increases deformity* or shows *disuse* of any part of his body or muscle groups.

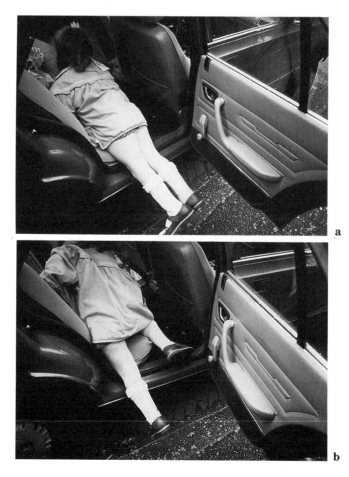

Fig. 4.1 a,b Child finding her own strategy of getting into a car; b is more desirable as she herself corrects spastic adduction of her legs.

Once a task is initiated by a child the therapist assists him to complete it. When unusual ways of performing a task are seen, then careful consideration is needed as these patterns do not always cause deformities or disuse and may be a variation of performance much like normal variations of motor function are acceptable in able-bodied people. When a child uses immature, pathological or biomechanically compensatory patterns which do cause deformity, blocking of further development or demand excessive energy then they are corrected and discouraged. However, these motor patterns may be the only ones possible for a child to achieve independence in a particular skill. It is then important to plan other motor activities in his day which use motor patterns to counteract the choice of his abnormal patterns for independence. Additional splinting and treatments are also added to counter undesirable motor patterns. Accepting abnormal motor patterns for independence in a skill depends on the age of a child as younger children have more potential for correction. The severity of the physical condition, the degree of intellectual impairment and the degree of visual disability lead to some compromise on the use of abnormal motor patterns for selected motor tasks.

Task analysis

In order to assess which movements and postures to improve, develop or discourage, a task analysis is made. The child's actions are compared with those in his age group and with those at an earlier stage of normal development. Task analyses include:

- A sequence of actions such as getting up from the floor through various postures (see Fig. 7.184). There is a sequence of actions for eating, drinking, washing and other daily tasks. There is a sequence of actions in using walking aids, wheelchairs and transfers or play equipment.
- The postural mechanisms at a particular developmental stage together with patterns of voluntary movements (synergies).
- The motor action and its related sensory, perceptual and cognitive areas. This involves analysing where a child looks and what he hears, smells, tastes and touches during the motor action. At the same time, he senses what he is doing in both movement and postural control (vestibular input and proprioception). Finally, what he understands as the purpose of his action and all the senses which inform him of this.

The physiotherapist also contributes to the motor components of a task by considering how the following affect the quality of motor function:

- Ranges of joint motion.

- Muscle lengths and strength.
- Postural alignments including asymmetries.
- Deformities both fixed and unfixed.
- Involuntary movements, spasms or reflex reactions which interfere with motor function.

These aspects are discussed in Chapter 6 which covers assessment.

There are different viewpoints on the analyses of tasks not only among physiotherapists but also between professionals. It is therefore necessary for members of a team to share their views on a child they all know. Common ground between physiotherapists has been discussed in Chapter 3, in the sections on Synthesis of treatment systems and Treatment principles. Research on motor analyses progresses and therapists need to continue their studies so that better task analyses are developed in the future. Interdisciplinary studies and experience also add to better task analyses involving sensory, perceptual, cognitive and motor interactions.

Cues for learning

Cues for learning need to be clearly given in therapy. Each child will respond to different cues according to his stages of development and the presence of specific impairments. Cues are given for the starting position, during the action and for the final result of the action. A child needs to detect or be informed of any errors in his performance as well as his success (Winstein & Schmidt 1989).

Therapists may use sensory input, verbal guidance and rewards to help a child learn motor control. Experts in motor learning call such cues *feedback*; they are not only given by a therapist but are intrinsic to the child's own experience in actively performing any task.

An example of an approach which may be adapted to different individuals is:

(1) *Set the scene so that a child can actively manage* what he can on his own. This means modifying the environment by having non-slip mats, place mats, appropriate toys, sturdy furniture and equipment according to the child's size and providing adequate light and colour to encourage achievement. In this way a child's own action gives him feedback for learning. He senses errors so that he can correct them through his understanding of the task and how to move. The use of motor patterns *he* discovers is best for learning, provided they do not seriously increase his symptoms.

(2) *A therapist's hands can physically guide* a child through a whole task to demonstrate what is to be done and how to do it (Fig. 4.2). She must then immediately remove her hands at any time that a child takes over this action from her. This may be at the beginning, middle or in finishing the task.

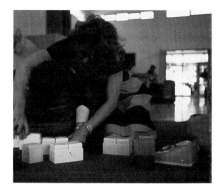

Fig. 4.2 Therapist's physical guidance through whole or part of motor task. Wedge positions child for hand function. If needed, set scene with playthings on floortable to activate head control and variation on hand use.

(3) *A therapist gives minimal support* to a child's body, shoulders or hips so that a task can be actively attempted and practised by a child. She may use equipment to support a child, as in the example given in Fig. 4.2.

(4) *Appropriate manual assistance or resistance* to a child's movements or stabilization of his head, body, hips and shoulders allows him to sense what to do and how to do it. Joint compression also alerts his sensory understanding of postural stabilization (fixation). The therapist's appropriate manual resistance also conveys to a child which body part to move and in which direction to move it. Other neuromuscular facilitation methods offer this as well.

(5) *Visual feedback* can inform a child of what he is to do and how he is doing it. Encourage him to look at his own body. Mirrors may help, though the reversed image may sometimes cause difficulties. His own observation of another child with cerebral palsy similar to him is most helpful. He may observe the therapist or his parent carrying out a task which he needs to learn. Observing others directly or on video can only be used for children who are able to imitate others. Thus severe visual impairment or severe learning impairments may make this impossible. Videos of themselves may be used by some children if they are not upset by seeing their inadequate performances.

(6) *Feedback with sounds, visual displays or vibration* can inform a child on the results of his actions. These biofeedback techniques may also be arranged to augment the most desirable motor patterns of posture and movement. However, like therapy 'exercises' they do not transfer to daily living if feedback on isolated actions is given (Mulder 1985). Babies and severely intellectually impaired children who cannot understand *cause and effect* are not able to use feedback. They have to learn that their movement created a sound or switched on a light.

Verbal guidance

This is only possible when a child understands words. It includes all or some of the following verbal instructions:

(1)   Informing a child what is going to happen or the purpose of the motor patterns, for example 'You are going to . . .'.
(2)   Suggesting the starting position, the movement or balance and commenting on the results of these motor patterns. This may be done together with physical guidance. For example when showing a child how to stand up from a chair, verbalize the skill by saying 'Keep your feet flat, go forward over your feet and stand up'.

However, it is usually best if minimal verbal guidance is used with all young children. Sometimes an operative word like 'step, step, step' or 'push, push, push' can be helpful. For many children, especially those who are multiply disabled, it is advisable to set the scene and physically guide or use clear gestures for communicating what is expected in a task. Also, use specialized (adaptive) equipment and toys. It is then best to be quiet and attentive as a child learns from his own experience. Quiet, encouraging looks at the task and glances towards a child avoid distractions from the task to what a therapist is saying. Such an approach encourages better focusing of that child's attention on the task.

Comments on the results of a child's efforts may not always be necessary if he clearly understands that he has achieved what he has set out to do. Motivation can be maintained by phrases such as 'you sat nice and straight' or 'you stretched your elbows well'. This provides the feedback of information and praise so that the task can be learnt.

Remember: care needs to be taken that physical guidance and words do not themselves distract a child. A child with visual impairment or multiple disabilities may become attracted to a therapist's touch or speech rather than keep his attention on the task to be learnt. One needs to avoid a child becoming passive and dependent on your physical guidance or *facilitation method*. It is wise to remove your hands as soon as possible.

Rewards

Although children can gain intrinsic reward in their own achievement of a task there are those who have such profound impairments that they warrant additional rewards which are extrinsic. Many teachers recommend giving a child with profound intellectual impairment a reward *immediately after* he has completed a task or even *the intention* to try to do it. Smiles, words of approval and of information may not be understood. Very basic rewards which do not depend on language or social development are suggested. There are many possibilities and each child is observed to discover what he prizes most as satisfaction. This may be food, juice, music or lights. A variety of tactile stimuli such as stroking, patting, cuddling, blowing on his face and vibration may please him particularly. The goals for a child must be tangible so that he can be rewarded, rather than fail to achieve goals well out of his range of abilities. It is important to observe when a child has had too much of the same reward and become bored with it. This applies to all children who enjoy the incentives of a variety of toys and play during daily tasks. We continually use our imagination to find satisfying rewards for children.

Apparent rewards of 'good boy', a hug and other social praise should not be used indiscriminately as for example, when a child is not doing anything constructive such as slumped in a chair or carrying out undesirable movements or mannerisms. This does not help learning and confuses a child as to what adults expect from him.

Natural rewards of enthusiasm and delight, together with clear information on what a child has struggled to achieve or tried to initiate are recommended. When basic rewards need to be used these are decreased as a child with profound learning disabilities learns and retains the achievement of a motor task (Williams 1978; Presland 1982).

Older children and young children who can appreciate it may be given a progress chart with ticks for abilities gained, or collect stars or tokens for achievement. They are also rewarded when their friends, classmates and their family members approve their hard work and specific achievements.

Practice and experience

In the next chapter the collaborative learning outlines ways of sharing the practice of a motor task with others assisting a child's development. Practice of a motor task incorporated into activities used by teachers, playgroup workers and family members is planned with them. A motor function is also practised on its own. The stages of learning are as follows:

(1) A consistent way in which postural control, postural alignment and movements are first practised so that some ability can be initiated and developed.

(2) In the therapy session a child may have tried out various different motor patterns to accomplish his goal and improved on them with a therapist's suggestions. When his own strategies were unsuccessful he will have been shown alternative patterns by his therapist. The successful patterns are those that will be practised so that they are consolidated. Whenever possible, the motor patterns discovered as successful for a child's purpose by that child are used. They may be unusual but not deforming nor increasing symptoms of motor dysfunction.

(3) Once consistency of practice has led to abilities, these are used in a variety of situations. A child is encouraged to use his motor function to explore inside and outside his home and school. He rolls, crawls or walks on different surfaces indoors and outdoors. Surfaces may be stationary at first, but moving for later motor control. This may happen when a child is taken on visits to shops, the zoo, the countryside and other places for his education as well as for his motor experiences. During these visits, time and patience need to be given so that he can use his movements and balance as he acquires sensory, perceptual and cognitive experiences. Various play experiences with sand, water, snow and many other materials are at first presented so that he uses his motor abilities or emerging abilities in play. Control of posture, movements and the use of his hands develops further during his own spontaneous exploration.

(4) It is best to develop and practise a task in a child's familiar environment. This offers him well known clues for learning motor function. When home visits or school visits are difficult, then a clinic or centre needs to create situations similar to those known by a child so that transfer of motor function learning can be achieved.

(5) The training of the motor components of posture and movement needs to happen at home either following or preceding their use in the whole motor function or daily living activity. In this way training motor components is not reserved for a clinical session in one venue and use of these components in their meaningful context in another venue. Training and practice of components are only necessary if these need to be separated due to the complexity of particular tasks. To help learning a child needs to understand the relevance of components to the whole task, as outlined in Chapter 5.

A word of caution: a child should not be made to feel that unless he is achieving a motor skill he will not be loved. Outside the therapy session he needs to feel loved and appreciated for the person he is whether he is working hard or not. There are many ways of building this attitude into relationships with a child.

Summary

Learning motor function needs to be integrated with the purpose or meaning of such motor function to a child. Consideration needs to be given to the following aspects of learning a motor function, either on its own or within a daily activity:

(1) Developing a child's attention.
(2) Discovering a child's own goals and strategies and following this lead.

(3) Analysing the task for learning for each child.

(4) Giving cues for learning what a child is going to do, how he performs and the results of what he does.

(5) A child's own actions and results of them provide him with sensory information for learning a task.

(6) Verbal intructions are usually minimal but are useful in children who understand them.

(7) There is intrinsic reward in achieving the task itself. However, external rewards may also be incentives for individuals.

(8) Practice is necessary to develop motor function. It needs first to be consistent and then within a variety of situations. A variety of movement experiences helps to reinforce motor learning.

Chapter 5
A Collaborative Learning Approach

Working with parents

Today, therapists recognize the importance of working with the mother of each child. Yet mothers become both physically and emotionally exhausted with caring for their children with disabilities, the rest of the family and possibly their own work outside the home. Many therapists have therefore also shared their programmes with fathers and other adults in a child's family. Not only are they a ready-made team, but their participation helps them feel of value to a child with a disability.

Rosenbaum *et al.* (1992), in their studies of components of care for children with disabilities, found that 'parental involvement' in decisions about their child 'reduces stress and personal worries'. This was stated at the top of the parents' list of components of care. I believe this applies to parent participation in therapy programmes.

In the last years I have been developing a style of working which involves a child along with his parents in a collaborative learning experience with a physiotherapist. All take responsibility in assessments, therapy and evaluations (Levitt & Goldschmied 1990). It is a creative learning process, not only for a child and his parents but also for any therapist. The therapist learns what the hopes and expectations of a child and his parents are and what they already know and can do. Using these resources, therapists are better able to draw on their technical expertise for a more relevant programme. The respect and trust given to what parents and child already understand and can manage develops their confidence. More positive relationships grow between parents, child and therapist. There is more motivation as parents and child respond positively to a therapist who appreciates their desires and their ideas for solving some of their own problems.

Collaboration with other adults

When considering parents as adult learners, I feel supported by the studies of workers such as Rogers (1983) and Knowles (1984) in adult education. It is useful to draw on their ideas, not only for parents but for other adults such as family members, other professionals and carers assisting a child's development. A physiotherapist or occupational therapist will grow both professionally and personally as she learns about the priorities and knowledge of these adults. She becomes better able to select and devise methods to suit individual adults involved with a child. She also gains information about various environments in which a child needs to function.

The collaborative learning approach

A child and his parents are offered:

- Opportunities to discover what they want to achieve.
- Opportunities to clarify what is needed for these achievements.
- Opportunities to recognize what they already know and can do.
- Opportunities to find out what they still need to learn and do.
- Participation in the selection and use of methods.
- Participation in the evaluation of progress.

Genuine participation in all these aspects by child and parents helps them feel more committed to the programme of work. It gives them some sense of control which decreases many of their anxieties and builds their confidence. They become more able and more willing to absorb ideas, information and practical suggestions from therapists.

This style of work with parents coincidentally tunes in with the views of Bailey & Simeonsson (1988) in the field of developmental disabilities. My focus is more on the neuromotor aspects and on a person with neurological conditions and his/her family. Bailey & Simmeonsson found in their many studies that parents and families want:

- Education and information.
- Parental training in skills to help their child.
- Emotional support.

This collaborative learning approach takes account of all these aspects. The studies of Sluys *et al.* (1993) call for more education of patients by their physiotherapists and my approach offers a response to this.

Opportunities to discover what parents and child want to achieve

Many parents are quick to say what their expectations from therapy are. Others want time to discuss this with their families. Some parents are unaccustomed to asserting what they want as they have anxieties and 'learned helplessness' (Greer & Wethered 1984; Seligman 1992). They may also sense that their therapist might be upset if they choose what therapy might focus on for *their* lives.

The therapist invites them to talk about a typical day in their lives by saying which daily activities they would like to improve further and

The therapist's specialized assessment   Once the motor and sensory components of a task have been observed by a therapist within a whole task, she decides how much more she needs to assess. She can then carry out more detailed assessments of muscle work, joint ranges and tone, postural mechanisms in all positions and other sensori-motor details. However, the advantage of first seeing all these separate aspects within a whole task reveals many ideas which challenge the accuracy of only using such separate examinations.

The tasks have been chosen by the parent or child and are being performed by a motivated person. Results of such an assessment tend to be more positive. There is interaction between all aspects of a task so that ability in one component activates any residual ability in another component. In my experience tests of reflexes may be abnormal if carried out in isolation, but if observed within the context of parent–child interactions during daily activities the assessment shows a more positive result. For example, a grasp reflex becomes immediately modified as a baby places her hand on her mother's breast during feeding; an assymetrical tonic neck response or a Moro reaction may be overcome as a child puts both her arms around her father's neck or holds her head up in eye-to-eye contact during activities (Levitt 1986).

Therapists will also discover the *task specificity* (Carr & Shepherd 1987) of muscle work and postural control. Assessments on the couch may or may not transfer into other positions or motor functions. For example, shoulder girdle muscles may work well in crawl position but not in a muscle test on the couch. Back extensors may be well activated in prone but not in sitting or standing. Extension of the elbow is greater when a child reaches out for a desired object than when tested with the conventional 'stretch your elbow' in muscle tests. Kerr (1992) refers to recent developments in physiology where activation of a muscle depends on the mechanical actions of other muscles acting around a joint.

Records are now made of:

- The priorities of parents and of a child: *ultimate aims.*
- What parents and child can already do: *baseline abilities.*
- What parents and child still need to achieve: *immediate aims* (see Chapters 4 and 6).

It may be easier to record the abilities and needs in a video. A framework is devised so that the same scenes are checked when evaluations are made. A set time for evaluation may be arranged so that the immediate aims or *behavioural objectives* are fully defined. This arrangement is also called a *contract* of long-term and short-term aims planned between parents, child and therapist.

Participation in the selection and use of methods

There is no sharp division between the assessments just described and methods. Many of the assessment methods become methods for training function. A therapist's addition of positioning, physical guidance and manual support become extended to include selection of equipment, orthoses and furniture, shoes and playthings.

As parent and child develop their confidence, they will share their own ideas with their therapist (Fig. 5.1). She always welcomes their ideas as they are showing an eagerness to take some responsibility in the programme and not become totally dependent on her. The therapist considers their suggestions and if inappropriate modifies them or shelves them for a later stage in a child's development. With any validation of the ideas of parents or child they become more able to cope with times when some of their ideas are incorrect. Clearly a therapist needs to become more flexible so she can be open to what parents and child offer. This means that she cannot stick rigidly to any system of therapy.

As with a child, a parent is first observed practising a method of training her/his child, then guided physically or verbally by the therapist to improve that method. Details are added according to what each parent can absorb and manage. Each parent also has their own pace of learning and some need many more repetitions of a method than others. We avoid overwhelming a parent with a 'mountain of knowledge and tasks'. This may exhaust them and disrupt family life creating additional feelings of inadequacy (Featherstone 1981; Hinojusa 1990; Ross & Thomson 1993).

Special physiotherapy techniques Once a parent has some confidence in methods for the familiar, everyday tasks in child care, they can add selected physiotherapy techniques. Some parents are intimidated by unusual techniques whereas others overdo them. They believe or want to believe that these strange techniques are 'magical treatments' and overdo them at the expense of developing their natural parenting abilities and positive relationships with their child. It is these relationships which are fundamental to real progress. Exercises such as ranges of motion,

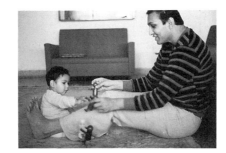

Fig. 5.1 There is pleasurable interaction between this father and his child as the child's postural control with hand function is being developed. Father chose to use his feet to assist his child in symmetrical weight bearing on hips and weight shifting from side to side or forwards and backwards during play.

stretchings, specific balance training and strengthening exercises may be carried out in a didactic style which parents may have observed in a physiotherapist treating their child or perhaps treating some other person with another medical condition. A study by Kogan *et al.* (1974) found that mothers acting as therapists interacted negatively with their children. This was not the experience of von Wendt *et al.* (1984), who found positive interactions by well supported parents.

Any negative behaviour need not happen if we first set the scene as described above and we find methods within play activities. For example, a child's postural mechanisms and movements are developed on his parent's lap, when being carried and handled during all daily activities and play (Figs 5.2 and 5.3). A child's spine and limbs can be stretched and moved within positioning for daily tasks as well as in water and during

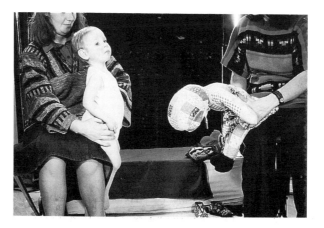

Fig. 5.2   Therapist showing tilt reaction facilitation on a doll so that this mother can interact with her child on her lap playing a 'see-saw' game. The position of the adult's hands on the child's hips rather than on the trunk is important.

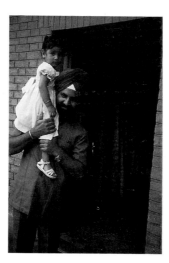

Fig. 5.3   A child developing postural control on her father's shoulders in playful activity.

musical rhythms and action songs. When a mother also assists a child to enjoy his body parts which are being kissed, tickled and touched by her as well as moved to her song, then she also develops a more positive view of her child's body. This pleasure in both mother and child contributes to their developing relationship in a creative way. It is important to develop parenting abilities at the same time as promoting a child's function and methods can be found to do this (Fig. 5.4). This also avoids an increased dependency and excessive demands on a therapist for 'magical treatments'. Parents need to recognize that their handling of their children is as important as special treatment sessions.

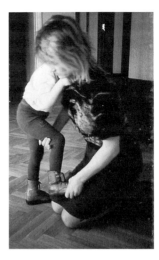

Fig. 5.4 Learning early balance on one foot during dressing and undressing, washing or drying with body closeness between mother and child.

Participation in the evaluation of progress

Throughout the therapy sessions it is reasuring for all to know how well they are progressing. Parent and child are asked to report on any new achievements based on the original assessments. They may have gained more of the steps in a sequence of actions in a daily activity or more postural control, more postural alignment or more hand use in their child.

Improvements from a child's baseline abilities can be recorded on video, with graphs or in written records. Professionals use their own recording techniques discussed in Chapter 6. These special methods as well as results of consultants' special tests need to be explained to parents and, when understanding is available, to a child.

Modifications of methods may then be made or new methods added for future progress. Equipment is checked together with parents to confirm correct size and function. The relevance of equipment to a child's home and lifestyle as well as acceptance of their aesthetic aspects is a continuing assessment with parents and child.

Behaviourial progress It is essential to comment on the progress of child and parent in their development of confidence, motivation, communication skills and personal relationships. It is after all not only functional gains that are important, but how much more viable life becomes for parents and child as a result.

Parent–child interaction

When familiar daily activities are used in the programme, a therapist is able to see a parent and child functioning together. As Winnicott (1964) points out 'there is no such thing as a baby, only a baby with someone else'. During these daily activities there is normally mutual pleasure between mother or father and child. However, a child with disabilities gives unusual communications as clues for a parent to know how to parent such a child. If a child has a floppy head, a visual problem or hypertonus this is not only a worry from a functional viewpoint but interferes with a child's response to a parent. Such a child cannot initiate communication with his head and eyes, hands or body to indicate his wants. Without head or trunk control a child cannot turn away from his parents to show when he has had too much stimulation and may become irritable. Parents may find their child hypersensitive to touch, difficult to cuddle or exhibiting unexpected startles of distress. It is easy for parents already unsure of their parenting abilities to feel rejected and anxious. The natural expertise of a therapist may make them feel more inadequate. There are, of course, other parents who are especially responsive to their child and discover many subtle cues of communication from their child. They can clarify for a therapist what their child's body communications and sounds mean.

It is essential that during the joint assessments of feeding, dressing, bathing, playing and other tasks, the therapist points out that:

- A child's unusual body actions, hypersensitivity or increase in stiffness is due to the cerebral palsy and not to poor parenting.
- A child's fears, apathy, hyperactivity or poor concentration are due to the cerebral palsy and not to poor parenting.

Enabling a parent to position a child well, to handle him and modify his neurological symptoms will improve not only motor function and daily activity but also communication and relationships. It is not just correct handling but a positive reciprocal interaction between parent and child that is being promoted (Figs 5.5 and 5.6a,b; see also Figs 5.1–5.4 for parent–child interaction).

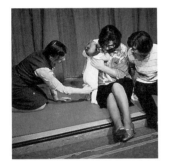

Fig. 5.5 Physiotherapist enabling a mother and her key person to learn how to activate early standing with close body contact as support.

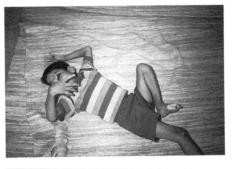

Fig. 5.6a Child with athetoid quadriplegia in supine.

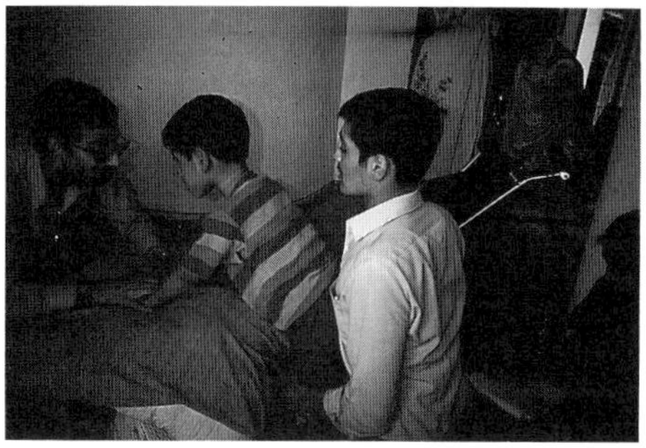

Fig. 5.6b Parent and child interact, promoting symmetrical standing leaning on both arms and so enabling the child to master his symptoms.

Helping a child to learn motor control

This is discussed in Chapter 4. The therapist makes sure that a parent develops these behaviours to reinforce a child's learning. Points to note are:

- Wait for a child's initiation for a motor action and follow his lead.
- Wait for a child's response to the parent's initiation of an activity.
- Adjust a task so that a child can experience some success.
- Find ways to alert and maintain a child's attention.
- Show appreciation for a child's small and large achievements.
- Grade sensory input so that a child is not overstimulated.
- Make appropriate demands on a child so he needs to make some effort to achieve a task without excessive increase in hypertonus, athetoid motion, tremors or startles and spasms.
- Give time for the gradual development of parent–child relationships and be patient with oneself as a parent learning to interact with an unusual child. Many parents have *their own ways of managing* which therapists must acknowledge, especially when cultural differences also exist.

Observation of parent and child interaction

There are psychologists and psychotherapists who are specialized in observing mother and baby interactions and the building of optimal relationships for a child's positive development (Stern 1985). There is increasing research effort on interactive styles of mothers with children with disabilities, some of which shows such mothers as being more directive as their children take fewer interactive turns with a parent (Hanzlik 1990). When a physiotherapist or occupational therapist assesses a child together with his parent, she can draw on the studies of psychologists or work closely with such a specialist on the team.

The therapist therefore observes not only the movements and postures which form the daily activities but also those that speak of the relationship between parent and child, and, between child and therapist. She informally notices the body language of how a mother and child look at each other, touch and move together. She notices how their bodies mould towards or away from each other. A child may initiate taking turns or need encouragement to do so in movement, eye contact or sounds and speech. The upright posture not only develops postural control but better communication and alertness. The way a parent supports and especially removes manual support demonstrates his/her anxiety and ability to trust a child to function alone. The parent's willingness to follow their child's lead and wait for their child's slow achievement can be very difficult for them.

The therapist needs to include such interactions in the therapy methods and may have to avoid methods which decrease positive interplay between parent and child. The therapist herself also models how to play, feed, dress, enable a child to move and enjoy these and other activities. However, care is always taken to make parents feel as competent as possible at their stage of learning. Information is regularly given on the neurological symptoms which can be modified to enhance communication and speech therapists can offer much in these areas. As a child is enabled to make a choice to communicate he will be more participant in this collaborative therapy approach (see Chapter 6).

Emotional support

It is clear that therapy is not just 'a bag of tricks' to increase a child's motor function or independent daily skills. A therapist is not only showing practical ideas but needs to give time for listening to the worries of a parent. However, she is always balancing her time for the parent and for the child. Listening and observing a child's facial expressions and body language tells her not only about the appropriate pace of work with a child but his emotional needs in general. When listening to a parent's or child's anxieties, a therapist need not immediately reassure them. It is a therapist's empathetic and attentive listening which serves them best. She needs to repeat back to each of them what she has heard them say and only later clarifies what she can do to help.

Therapists become aware of a variety of underlying anxieties in individual parents. A parent may be experiencing a complex mixture of emotions such as despair, anger, disapointment, frustration or guilt. This not only varies from parent to parent but in the same parent at different periods in their life with their child. Hall (1984), among others, perceives such emotions as part of the grieving process related to loss of the expected normal baby. There is hardly time for parents to work through this grief as they feel pressure to accept the very different child who is alive and may be making great demands on them physically and emotionally.

Therapists face a difficult situation in which their offer of help can make a parent feel more helpless. Some parents may then become more dependent on a therapist and burden her with excessive demands. Others resent their dependency, becoming angry that they should need professionals to show them how to parent their child. This anger can also be directed at the very professionals who are doing their best for such parents. Either way, a therapist needs to grow in maturity and they become the 'patient ones' rather than the patients. To do this therapists benefit from their own support groups and sensitive support from others in a team. This support is essential to maintain therapists' energy, understanding and motivation (Greer & Wethered 1984; Chapter 1 in Levitt 1984; Price 1991).

When a parent is particularly stressed, taking excessive time and energy from a physiotherapist or other professional, then this needs to be discussed with the team or with a qualified psychotherapist, family therapist or specialized counsellor. The therapist will gain guidance on how best to manage such a parent and if *and* how to refer such parents for professional help from psychotherapy.

The collaborative approach described changes the situation of a professional being the helper and the parent the helpless one to that of more equal partnership. The therapist therefore is not placed in any position where her help is rejected which may understandably upset her, possibly inviting anger. The parent learns to ask for help instead of just receiving it. Parents who find it difficult to accept help may be able to do so in a more collaborative situation with therapists.

Teamwork with parents

The example of the collaborative learning approach can be carried out best with the therapist as the key person or primary interventionist. This has the advantage of developing an ongoing relationship between therapist and child along with his parents and other members of the family. Parents find that visits from one professional is more desirable than from a stream of experts. One person can coordinate the habilitation programme and avoid contradictory advice from different sources. This is particularly helpful in community work.

The key person will be designated by a team of professionals who will support her with their assessments and selection of ideas to suit the aims of parents and child. The key person will learn from the team when specialized assessments and advice are necessary and when any specialized 'hands-on' sessions are indicated. This applies to any other key worker designated by a team, who is also compatible with parents and child. He/she will judge the frequency of home visits so that dependency is not generated by them (McConachie 1986).

This type of teamwork is called the *transdisciplinary* model. There can also be an *interdisciplinary* model in which collaboration with parents can take place between each professional such as physiotherapist, occupational therapist, speech therapist and teacher. Each professional will integrate the ideas of the others into her sessions with child and parents. When professionals work as a multidisciplinary team then such integration is rarely attempted as each professional carries out her own assessments and therapy or teaching sessions in the area of his or her discipline.

AN INTEGRATED APPROACH

In both the transdisciplinary model and interdisciplinary model, or combinations of both, professionals working with a child and the parents need to carefully learn the following:

(1)   Which postures and movements, including patterns of locomotion, to encourage so that a child develops them through practice in all environments.
(2)   Which undesirable motor and other behaviours to discourage.
(3)   Which positions make it easier for a child to see, hear, move and communicate.
(4)   How to prevent and correct deformities.
(5)   Which sensory, perceptual and cognitive experiences to encourage.
(6)   Which aids, equipment or orthoses to use to facilitate a child's function.
(7)   How to lift and carry a child so that he participates and corrects his neuromotor problems, and how this is done to protect the backs of the adults.
(8)   Which toys, playthings and recreational activities are specially recommended.

All these areas of specialized information for the individual child are interwoven by a team of collaborative adults so that a whole programme is shared with a child. In Chapter 10, such collaboration is outlined when a child is in a peer group.

Teamwork is facilitated in many ways. For example:

- Staff conferences in small or large meetings.
- Staff meetings may or may not include parents, depending on the agenda and parent's availability.
- Informal discussions with team members including parents.
- Visits to one another's workplace.
- Combined sessions with different therapists, with teachers, with health visitors or with social workers.
- Assessment by a number of professionals together with parents can be arranged using a one-way window so that the key person and child are alone together in a room. A parent may be in the room or watching with other professionals to learn about their child's actions and behaviour. Parents can then talk easily as they are not in front of their child and their comments add to everyone's insight. It is important to know whether a child's behaviour with professionals is typical or different from that at home (Newson 1976).

Parents' health

Physiotherapists are well trained to advise parents on where to learn relaxation methods and to care for their backs and general health. Information on parent support groups, special organizations and respite child care needs to be obtained for parents who want this. Financial advice may be needed by some parents and moments of crises of various kinds will be handled by social workers and the team. Unless the priorities of parents and families are appreciated, then attention to physiotherapy and occupational therapy advice and programmes may be difficult for parents to manage (Fox 1975; Tarran 1981). Parents need to have their worries appreciated and respected or they cannot give full attention to the suggestions of therapists.

Siblings

Although a therapist is busy with a child she needs to acknowledge the feelings of his siblings as well. Their normal rivalries are difficult to handle, especially when their brother or sister with disabilities receives so much extra attention. It is wise not to shoulder them with responsibilities for any treatment of their sibling. Although they may respond to their mother's need 'for an extra pair of hands', this should not be overdone. Brothers and sisters may respond to play activities which are therapeutic for the child with disabilities. They may invent their own games together (Levitt 1994).

Simeonsson & McHale (1981) found many individual reactions in siblings which may be positive in many respects, especially if they are not overburdened and given their own lives to lead as well.

Summary

A collaborative learning approach involves a therapist in a joint venture with a child and his parents. It can be used with other family members and with colleagues in a team. It is a radical departure from the traditional model in which a therapist takes full responsibility for assessments, treatment plans, use of methods and evaluation. Instead, all this is shared with parents and a child who can understand this.

Emotional aspects are outlined in relation to parent–child interaction, as well as therapist–child and therapist–parent interactions. The education, and the needs of parents and their priorities are given attention as well as care for their health. Therapists also deserve support in their own groups and teams. The collaborative learning model enables a therapist to develop both professionally and personally and learn to knit together ideas from counselling, communication skills and the study of human relationships.

Brazelton (1976) suggested that

'the success of any intervention programme should be measured not only by the child's development but by increased family comfort, decrease in the divorce rate, lower incidence of behaviour problems in siblings ... perhaps by pretty soft signs but they may be a lot more important as measures of effectiveness of intervention than is a rise in IQ or increased motor capacity on the part of the child'.

Chapter 6
Assessment for Therapy and Daily Function

Approach to assessment

In the last chapter it was shown how the therapist's assessment needs to grow out of her collaboration with the child and his parents and that assessment of separate aspects of posture, movement and sensation have to be observed within the context of whole functions. This chapter reviews the specific assessments by a physiotherapist and refers to the links with occupational therapy.

PURPOSE OF ASSESSMENT

A therapist needs to gather observations of a child in the following situations, as well as handling the child herself:

- As a child enters and leaves the room and while on his parent's lap or among attractive toys on the floor.
- During the activities being assessed as described in the last chapter.
- During a child's spontaneous behaviour at home, school or in the playground.

OUTLINE OF A THERAPIST'S OBSERVATIONS

These are made during the joint assessment with parents and in any *hands-on* assessment and treatment by a therapist.

(1) *Behaviour*   Observe whether a child is alert, apathetic, irritable or fearful in a session or during particular activities. A child may become fatigued easily, make undue effort or show discomfort during an activity.

(2) *Communication*   Observe how child and parent interact. Find out whether a child initiates or responds with gestures, sounds, hand or finger pointing, eye pointing or uses words and speech.

(3) *Attention span*   What catches a child's attention? How does a parent assist him to maintain attention and what distracts him?

(4) *Understanding*   Does a child follow suggestions to move or promptings to act? What does he appear to understand?

(5) *Position*   Which position does he choose to be in and can he get

into that position on his own or with help? Observe if a parent can place him in position and if he participates in any way. His limbs and head may move more easily in some positions than in others. Involuntary movements may be decreased in some positions.

(6) *Postural control and alignment* Observe how much parental support is given and check a child's own ability in postural stabilization and counterpoising in all postures. Check whether a child bears more weight on one side of his body, or on one hand or foot. A child may collapse to one side, twist to one side or tilt and turn his head to one side.

(7) *Use of limbs and hands* Observe limb patterns in changing or going into a position as well as using them in a position. There may be excessive flexion, extension or rotation in one part of the range. Observe whether one or both hands are used, type of grasp and release. Accuracy of reach and hand actions also indicates a possible visual problem. Observe any involuntary movements, tremors or spasms which interfere with actions.

(8) *Sensory aspects* Observe a child's use of vision, hearing, of touch, smell and temperature in relevant tasks. Does he enjoy particular sensations? Notice whether he enjoys being moved or having his position changed.

(9) *Form of locomotion* On entering the room observe how a child is carried, uses a wheelchair or uses walking aids. During the session create interest which motivates him to roll, creep, crawl, bottom shuffle or walk to where a daily activity is to be carried out. A child may have unusual ways of getting about such as dragging himself along his stomach, along his back, *bunny hopping* on both knees, *running headlong* and other gaits.

(10) *Deformities* Observe any recurring positions of the whole child as well as of parts of his body in all postures and in the movements he uses. This observation is checked with passive ranges of motion.

Note in Chapter 7 the details of motor assessment are given at each developmental stage under the headings of common problems, abnormal postures, abnormal gait and basic arm and hand patterns for all levels of development. The parent and child interactions are informally observed as outlined in Chapter 5

TEAMWORK AND THE INFLUENCE OF OTHER DISABILITIES

The therapist will need a comprehensive assessment from a team (see Chapter 1). She will learn from the different professionals what modifications to make for specific visual, hearing and sensory impairments. She will adjust her communication with a child in relation to any speech and language difficulties and find out what communication systems are being used, for example Paget, Makaton or Bliss. If a child has perceptual problems then adaptations will be advised for these difficulties during activities.

General points to remember for assessments

- Keep sessions within the bounds of a child's concentration.
- Have an unhurried atmosphere. Keep it playful if possible.
- Make your expectations of a child as clear as possible.
- Keep the sequence of specific assessment to suit a child's preference, though recording will be made more systematically.
- Have easy, successful actions of a child interspersed with difficult tasks.
- Avoid undressing a child until he is happy about this.
- Begin treatment of some motor functions at the first assessment so parents and child go away with something to practise. Assessments merge into methods used and re-assessments.
- Assessments take from one to four sessions depending on each child. Time is also needed for a child who is unhappy about a new environment, a new professional and the new experience of being assessed in a different style.

Value of assessment

- *To plan a therapy programme* which includes special neuromuscular techniques, selection of equipment and advice to parents and others caring for the child.
- *To assess progress* which may lead to continuation, modification, changes or sometimes periodical stopping of specific therapy sessions.
- *To add observations* to the diagnostic picture. The therapist should also add to the diagnostic information as her specific assessments before *and* during therapy involve long periods of time and close contact with the child and his family. Information may be revealed to the therapist which may not have been obvious in the shorter consultations with the different consultants.

Assessment methods

These vary from centre to centre and work is still in progress to find universal assessments which are objective, reliable, valid and relevant to practical therapy.

This chapter offers a framework for assessment for practical therapy. As a synthesis of various systems is used in therapy it is not possible to use assessment methods from any one approach. However, the common factor in all treatment systems is that they all ultimately aim at the child's independent motor function. Therefore a functional assessment is used (see the illustration of developmental levels in the Appendix). In addition

grading will reveal no progress when the child has really achieved the beginning of a new skill or partially achieved it. In these cases therapists and parents have also found that by giving some additional assistance, these skills can be fully achieved by the child and ease the life of the child and the family. *No progress* is not only inaccurate but discouraging to everyone in these slow developing children. Various gradings exist in different centres. I do not use those that chart any assistance as this is difficult to measure, remember or record without long descriptions of *how much, where given* and *for how long* within the duration of the motor act. Assessment is primarily to find out how the child copes without any help. Assistance may be recorded as part of the advice for parents and others caring for the child. It is of course essential to record this information in the minds of those caring for the child by demonstration.

Grading may be:

(0)   No ability.
(1)   Beginning, partially achieved, unreliable, insecure, momentary.
(2)   Reliably achieved, efficient.

It is obvious that the items on the developmental channels will be assessed and graded so that the therapist finds out what he cannot do (0) and what he can do (1, 2). Grading 3 can include *reliable with good pattern* as opposed to *very* abnormal pattern in 2. Abnormal performance or pattern is particularly difficult to grade on a chart. It is, however, essential to have a grading or some record for therapy and for progress. A child may not only progress by obtaining a new ability but also by improving *the way* he carries out his existing abilities. This may be anecdotal or on video.

Therapists must observe the child's head, trunk, arms, legs in all motor activities during assessment and during therapy. Depending on the child and the therapist's experience much time may be needed.

This information may be written out or an attempt to grade this information may be made in general groups of severe, moderate and mild. This is possible if the categories are described in a list of instructions but it is seldom strictly accurate. If grading includes 'very abnormal' and 'good' therapists will be accurate in this more obvious range. There are other tools for observation and recording which include films, video-tapes, various photographic methods, notation methods such as that of Benesh, Laban and others, electromyography and other more specific methods for specific problems of weight bearing, spasticity, joint range, gait pattern and weakness (Holt 1965; Holt *et al.* 1974). Gait Laboratories offer useful information on these aspects in individual cases. Figure 6.1 shows a clinical gait analysis.

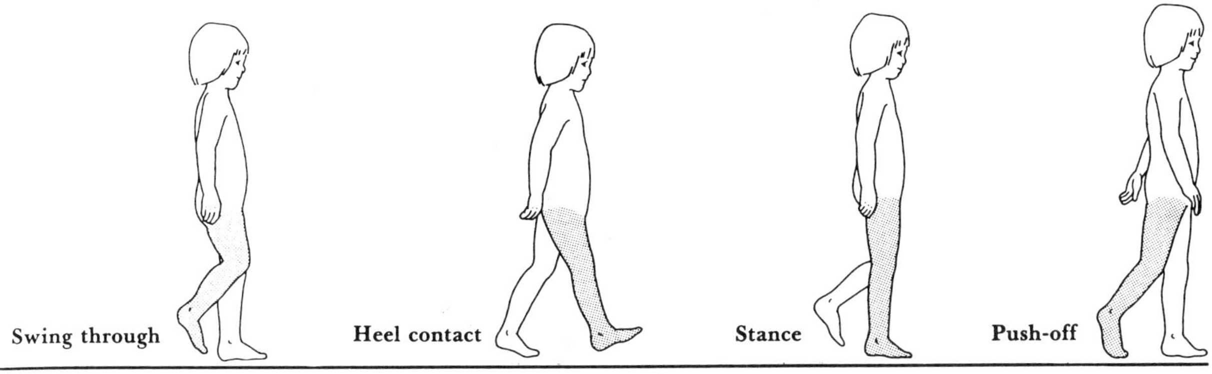

Swing through — **Heel contact** — **Stance** — **Push-off**

Swing through		Heel contact	Stance	Push off
Elements:	initial swing mid swing terminal swing	initial contact/strike loading	midstance	terminal stance pre-swing
Swing 40%			stance 60%	
Head	Erect forward/down shift	Erect arrest forward/down shift	Erect	Erect forward/downward shift
Trunk	Erect lateral shift to left	Erect lateral shift to right	Erect lateral shift to right	Erect lateral shift to left
Pelvis	Rotates from back to forward on right Lateral tilt down, right	Forward rotation right Lateral tilt up right	Level Lateral tilt up right	Rotates back as contralateral left rotates forward Lateral tilt down right
Hip	Flexion 20°	Flexion 30°	Extension	Extension 10°
Knee	Flexion 70° changing to extension	Full extension, semiflex on loading.	Full extension	Extension becomes 30° flexion
Ankle	Plantarflex to neutral	90°	90°	Neutral change to plantarflex to swing.
Arms	Right swing back, left forward	Right back swing, left forward swing.	Midway	Right forward, left back.
Examples of abnormal gaits	Failed ballistic swing giving short stride. Foot drag. Failed left stance giving quick limp onto right. Overflexed swing (high step). Abnormal pelvic tilts and rotations. Circumduction.	Toe contact, whole foot contact; swivel on toe while loading. Forward shift abnormal, continues as *run* or backward lean. Unstable. Hip flexion – hyperextended knee. Hip flex – lordosis – pelvic tilt. Pelvic retraction; abnormal rotation.	On toe; pronation, equinovarus. Hip, knee flexion: overflexed ankle. Hyperextended knee. Excessive hip internal rotation/external rotation; adducted/abducted pelvic retraction. Excessive pelvic tilt up. Antero-posteriorly tilts excess. Unstable. Fleeting stance phase. No lateral shift.	Absent phase and *fall* on to left excessive lateral shift or forward minimal hip extension: hip rotates overflexion all joints: no plantar extension. Pelvic drop excessive on right. Equinovarus or valgus *push off*. Abnormal hip adduction. Abnormal posture and patterns as seen in *swing through*.

Note In all phases of gait kyphosis, lordosis, scolioses, abnormal head position, abnormalities of arm postures/swing may be present.

Fig. 6.1 Right leg gait analysis (child over 2 years of age). Note also: speed, base, rhythm and step sizes, endurance (distance), EMG. (Source: Levitt S., 1984.)

Abnormal performance and deformity

Observation of abnormal performance is the primary but not only observation of abnormal positions of the joints in posture and movement. These are the unfixed or fixed deformities. Specific examinations of the child's joints and muscles should also be made to check whether there is a fixed or unfixed deformity. Fixed deformity due to structural change, leg length or soft tissue contraction will explain abnormal performance on a mechanical level. Unfixed deformity is more complicated. It changes with position of the body, spastic muscle length and pattern of active movements, *and* with a child's mood and the time of day.

EXAMINATION OF DEFORMITY

The therapist should obtain information on:

- *Structure of joints* especially subdislocation or dislocation of the hips, varus or valgus neck of femur, spinal vertebrae.
- *Inequality in the length of legs* but not so much in the arms, as far as function is concerned.
- *Joint range* Passive range of motion carried out slowly may detect fixed or unfixed deformity as well as tightness of muscle groups. Quick passive stretch detects *hypertonus*. Active range is also needed but has already been observed in the functional examination where it is of the greatest significance.

Passive range (figures and captions – Table 6.1)

Active range (Table 6.1)

Head and trunk flexion, extension, rotation observed during head raise in prone, supine, sitting, standing developmental channels.

Shoulder elevation, abduction, rotation, flexion and extension movements are observed during the functional examination of, say, creeping, reaching and other arm movements.

Elbow flexion and extension observed during child's reach to parts of his body or toys. Forearm pronation or supination affects flexion and extension, and must also be seen in isolation.

Wrist and hand will be observed during hand function development.

Hip flexion and extension will be observed during all functions. Also ask the child to lie supine, bend his hip and knee to his chest and touch his

Table 6.1 Assessment of joint range.

Assess:

Passive joint range: to demonstrate muscle length (extensibility, shortening), muscle tightness (spasticity, rigidity) and soft tissue tightness. Remember that muscle tightness (hypertonus) may or may not have full range of motion.
Degree of tightness or resistance to your passive motion, and where the greatest degree occurs in the range.
The difference between muscle and soft tissue tightness. Test *slowly*, use inhibitory techniques and sometimes anaesthetics to inhibit muscle tightness and reveal true contracture (fixed deformity).
Active joint range for range and ability to move and *not* as equivalent to muscle strength. Quality of muscle action should be noted. Strength and the opposing degree of tightness affect active range.

Note: different positions may affect range of motion in some cases. Check in supine, prone, sitting, sidelying, standing as well.

Hip flexor tightness – extension range
Bend one knee to chest. The other may flex off bed. Overcome this hip flexion by downward pressure on the front of the thigh: Check how far this can be over-come, and how much pressure is required.
or
Bend both knees to chest. Hold one bent and see how far the other can be stretched down to the bed.
Prone-hip extension is usually inaccurate because of pelvic-trunk compensation.

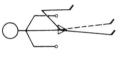
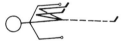

Hip extensor tightness – flexion range
Bend both hip and knee to chest. Note range and degree of extensor tightness.
Hip extensor tightness also revealed in knee flexor test for hamstrings below.

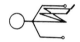

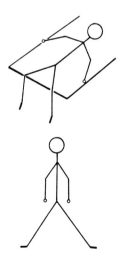

Hip adductor tightness – abduction range
Test in supine and in prone. Abduct hips with hips straight, knees bent. Abduct hips with hips and knees flexed. Abduct hips with hips and knees extended. These three procedures reveal tightness in different muscle groups and show which requires therapy and positioning; 50–80° is normal abduction with extended hips.

Table 6.1 Continued

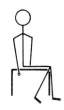

Hip adductor tightness – abduction range
Bring legs together and hips straight from *frog position* if present.

Hip rotator tightness – internal or external rotation
Assess with hip and knee flexed and extended. Rotate thigh inwards and outwards.

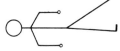

Knee flexor tightness – extension range
Bend one knee to eliminate hip flexion-lordosis and test the other. With hip at 90–100° fully extend that flexed knee.

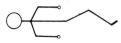

Straight leg lift also reveals tight hamstrings (flexor tightness at knees and extensor tightness at hips).

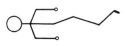

Press knees straight in lying supine or prone (limited range may be detected).

Knee extensor tightness – flexion range
Lying prone, flex the knee. If hip rises up into flexion, press hip down as far as possible to detect tightness of biceps femoris.

Sitting: flex knee for tightness of quadriceps.
Note any *high-riding* patella.

Table 6.1 Continued

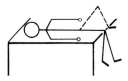

Lying knees flexed over edge of bed without lordosis. Bend one knee to counter lordosis and also eliminate hip flexor tightness (if present) with tests above.

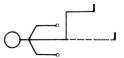

Foot plantar flexion tightness – dorsiflexion range
Bend hip and knee and dorsiflex foot by grasping heel and *avoiding* passive dorsiflexion in mid-foot. Hold dorsiflexion with knee straight.
Foot: inversion, eversion, plantarflexion tested with knee straight.

Note: keep pelvis level (stop antero-posterior tilt, lateral tilt) during assessments

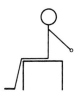

Shoulder flexor tightness – extensor range
Bring arm straight back.

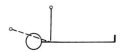

Shoulder flexor-adductor tightness – elevation range
Elevate arm forward and overhead.
Abduct and elevate arm.

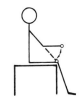

Shoulder rotations internal–external
Elbow flexor tightness – extension range
Slowly stretch *without* forcing elbow into extension with pronation and into extension with supination.

Elbow extensor tightness – flexion range
Bend elbow with pronation and test with supination.

Elbow pronation-supination

Carry out test with upper arm close to side of body.

Wrist flexion-extension

Wrist deviation radial and ulnar

Finger and thumb adduction and abduction

Finger and thumb flexion-extension

Remember to hold thumb at its base.

Head and trunk
Ranges rarely assessed unless torticollis or scoliosis is present.

Active ranges assessed as above but denotes action of antagonists overcoming tightness of agonists above. See also assessment within functional examinations.
Check: speed – rhythm – endurance of active assessments here and in functional assessments.
Note: Goniometry is measurement used for degrees of joint ranges.
Grade strength can be accurate only as: present, weak, strong.

Based on Andre-Thomas *et al.* (1960), Paine & Oppé (1966), Milani-Comparetti & Gidoni (1967), Prechtl (1977), Capute *et al.* (1978), Bobath (1980) and Illingworth (1980).

Table 6.2 Reflex reactions. A reflex conveys a stereotyped response to a stimulus. As responses vary in children the term reflex reaction is used.

Reflex reaction	Normal until	Stimulus	Response	Therapy
Sucking	3 months	Introduce a finger into mouth	Sucking action of lips and jaw	Train correct feeding
Rooting	3 months	Touch baby's cheek	Head turns toward stimulus	
Cardinal points	2 months	(1) Touch corner of mouth	(1) Bottom lip lowers on same side and tongue moves toward point of stimulation. When finger slides away, the head turns to follow	Desensitize face by child's own touch and other stimuli by therapist
		(2) Centre of upper lip is stimulated	(2) Lip elevates, tongue moves toward place stimulated. If finger slides along oronasal grove the head extends	
		(3) Centre of bottom lip is stroked	(3) Lip is lowered and tongue directed to site of stimulation. If finger moves toward chin, the mandible is lowered and head flexes	
Grasp	3 months	Press finger or other suitable object into palm from ulnar side	Fingers flex and grip object. (Head in mid-line during this test)	Weight bearing, stimuli over whole hand, hand opening in Development of hand function
Hand opening	1 month	Stroke ulnar border of palm and little finger	Automatic opening of hand	
Foot grasp	9 months	Press sole of foot behind the toes	Grasping response of feet	Weight bearing in Development of standing
Placing	Remains	Bring the anterior aspect of foot or hand against the edge of a table	Child lifts limb up to step onto table	Use in provoking early step
Primary walking (Automatic Walk: Reflex Stepping)	2 months	Hold baby upright and tip forward, sole of foot presses against table	Initiates reciprocal flexion and extension of legs	Weight bearing in Development of standing
Galant's trunk incurvation	2 months	Stroke back lateral to the spine	Flexion of trunk towards side of stimulus	Train trunk stability in Development of sitting and standing
Automatic sitting	2 months	Pressure is placed on the thighs and the head is held in flexion. Supine position.	Child pulls to sitting from supine	Train child's own rising in Development of sitting
Moro	0–6 months	Baby supine and back of head is supported above table. Drop head backwards, associated with loud noise	Abduction and extension of arms. Hands open. This phase is followed by adduction of the arms as if in an embrace	Train vertical head stability, use grasp, use prone position, use flexion position, shoulder fixation with grasp or hand support

Table 6.2 Continued

Reflex reaction	Normal until	Stimulus	Response	Therapy
Startle	Remains	Obtained by sudden loud noise or tapping the sternum	Elbow is flexed (not extended as in the Moro reflex) and the hand remains closed	Desensitize to noise by warning and experience
Landau	From 3 months to $2\frac{1}{2}$ years, strong	Child held in ventral suspension, lift head	The head, spine and legs extend. Extend arms at shoulders	Use in therapy to activate extensor muscles
	10 months	When the head is depressed	The hip, knees and elbows flex	
Flexor withdrawal	2 months	Supine; head mid-position, legs extended – stimulate sole of foot	Uncontrolled flexion response of stimulated leg (do not confuse with response to tickling)	Weight bearing, joint compression, knee splints and calipers in Development of standing
Extensor thrust	2 months	Supine; head, mid-oposition, one leg extended opposite leg flexed – stimulate sole of flexed leg	Uncontrolled extension of stimulated leg (do not confuse with response to tickling)	
Crossed extension	2 months	Supine; head, mid-position; legs extended – stimulate medial surface of one leg by tapping	Opposite leg adducts, extends, internally rotates and foot plantarflexes (typical scissor position)	
Asymmetrical tonic neck (ATNR) reaction	6 months, usually pathological	Patient supine; head in mid-position; arms and legs extended – turn head to one side	Extension of arm and leg on face side, or increase in extensor tone; flexion of arm and leg on skull side or increase in flexor tone	Use both arms together and train head in midline, use prone position, only encourage in severe older child
Symmetrical tonic neck (STNR) reflex	Rare and usually pathological	(1) Patient in quadruped position or over tester's knees – ventroflex the head (2) Position as above, dorsiflex the head	Arms flex or flexor tone dominates; legs extended or extensor tone dominates Arms extend or extensor tone dominates; legs flex or flexor tone dominates	See Prone development Correct weight bearing on hands and knees. If correct abnormal posture in all development then usually ignore the STNR
Tonic labyrinthine supine	Pathological	Patient supine; head in mid position; arms and legs extended. Test stimulus – is the position	Extensor tone dominates when arms and legs are passively flexed	See Development in supine; Development of sitting Overcomes excessive extension
Tonic labyrinthine prone *Reaction to prone*	3 months	Turn patient prone – head in mid-position. Test stimulus – prone position	Unable to dorsiflex head, retract shoulders, extend trunk, arms, legs	See Development in prone Overcomes excessive flexion
Positive supporting	3 months	Hold patient in standing position – press down on soles of feet	Increase of extension in legs. Plantarflexion, genu recurvatum may occur	See Development of standing Excessive anti-gravity response
Negative supporting	3–5 months	Hold in weightbearing position	Child 'sinks' astasia	See Development of standing

Table 6.2 Continued

Reflex reaction	Normal until	Stimulus	Response	Therapy
Neck righting	5 months	Supine, rotate head to one side, actively or passively	Body rotates as a whole in same direction as the head	See Development of rolling in supine Stimulate body rotative reactions
Associated reactions	Pathological	Have patient squeeze an object (with a hemiplegic, squeeze with uninvolved hand)	Clench of other hand or increase of tone in other parts of the body. Abnormal overflow	See Development of hand functions

Reflex reaction	Emerges at	Stimulus	Response	Therapy
Rising Labyrinthine head righting Vestibular righting (decrease of head lag)	2–6 months	(1) Hold blindfolded patient in prone position, in space, as head drops	Head raises to normal position, face vertical, mouth horizontal	For all reactions, see all sections on Developmental training in Chapter 7
		(2) As above in supine position	Head raises to normal position, face vertical, mouth horizontal	
	6 months	(3) Hold blindfolded patient in space – hold around pelvis, tilt to the side	Head rights itself to normal position, face vertical, mouth horizontal	
Optical	6 months	As above, no blindfold	As above	
Amphibian	4–6 months	Patient prone, head in mid-position, legs extended, lift pelvis on one side	Automatic flexion outward of hip and knee on same side	
(a) Body righting, derotative	4–6 months	Supine – rotate head or one knee one side, passively	Active derotation at waist, i.e. segmental rotation of trunk between shoulders and pelvis	
(b) Rotative	6–10 months	Rotate hip and knee or arm or head actively	Active segmented rotation (hyperactive at 10 months, cannot lie supine)	
Lift reaction (*not* the pathological lift reaction (Tardien))	5–6 months	Lift body through space	Head raises (lifts)	
Shoulder/pelvic girdle righting	3–6 months	Fix distal part(s) of limb	Rise up on to limb	

Postural fixation counterpoising (see the sections on developmental training in Chapter 7)

Tilt reactions

(a) Supine and prone	6 months	Patient on tiltboard. Arms and legs extended, tilt board to one side	Lateral curving of head and thorax, protective reaction in limbs accompany trunk reaction	

Table 6.2 Continued

Reflex reaction	Emerges at	Stimulus	Response	Therapy
(b) Four point kneeling	7–12 months	Patient in quadruped position, tilt toward one side	Lateral curving of head and thorax. Abduction-extension of arm and leg on raised side and protective reactions on lowered side may accompany this	
(c)		Tilt forward and back (antero-posteriorly)	Forward – head and back, flex. Backward – head and back, extend	
(d) Sitting	9–12 months	Patient seated on chair – tilt patient to one side. Tilt forward anteroposterior back	Head and thorax curve abduction-extension of arm and leg on raised side, other protective reactions may accompany this	
(e) Sitting		Tilt forward	Child extends head and back	
		Tilt back	Child flexes head and trunk	
(f) Kneel-standing	18 months	Patient in kneel-standing position, pull or tilt patient to one side	As above	See Chapter 7
(g) Standing	12–18 months	Patient in standing position. Tilt sideways. Tilt anteroposteriorly	Trunk as above	
Staggering reactions (see Saving from falling below)	12–18 months	(1) Move to left or to right side push or holding upper arm	Hopping, or step sideways to maintain equilibrium	
		(2) Move forward	Hopping, or step forwards to maintain equilibrium	
		(3) Move backwards	Hopping, or step backwards to maintain equilibrium or dorsiflex feet going on to heels	
Saving from falling	5–10 months	Prone – sudden tip downward Sitting – sudden tip downward Standing – sudden tip downward	Immediate extension of arms with abduction and extension of fingers to save and then prop the child	
	6–9 months	Standing – sudden tip sideways – one arm		
	9–12 months	Standing – sudden tip backwards – both arms		

Note motor patterns of the responses may be abnormal. This is *not* a chart for testing a child, but as background information for observation in function.

Based on Andre-Thomas *et al.* (1960), Paine & Oppé (1966), Milani-Comparetti & Gidoni (1967), Prechtl (1977), Capute *et al.* (1978), Bobath (1980) and Illingworth (1980).

plasters, splintage or bracing makes it possible for an *active* participation of other parts of the child's body or of the particular part of the body being corrected. Always assess how a child is positioned in special equipment and how he uses any aids to decide on their effectiveness.

Summary

(1) Assessment is essential for a therapy plan which is relevant to each child.

(2) Assessment methods must be selected in *direct* relationship to techniques of treatment. Such a practical approach is outlined in this chapter.

(3) Objective valid, reproducible assessments and records still need research.

(4) The practical assessment in this chapter includes a developmental functional assessment, examination of deformity (threatening or established), of daily living activities and equipment and can be used for checking progress.

(5) Additional assessments of communication, perception and play and social behaviour are also needed.

(6) The way in which you approach a child in assessment affects the information obtained.

Note: see Appendix for the Physical ability assessment guide and the Developmental levels illustrations.

Chapter 7
Treatment Procedures

MOTOR DEVELOPMENTAL TRAINING

ASSESSMENT AND TECHNIQUES

The chapters that follow are presented in relation to the assessment findings of *motor delay, abnormal performance* and *reflex reactions*. The assessment findings given are based on much clinical experience. However, there will still be individual problems which cannot all be included in one book.

DEVELOPMENTAL LEVELS AND TECHNIQUES

It is important to read the section on Developmental training in Chapter 3, the section on Developmental levels – Assessment and Therapy in Chapter 6, and all of Chapter 4 on the motor learning processes to understand how to follow and modify normal developmental levels for motor delay and especially motor disorder.

In practice, follow each channel of development for prone, supine, sitting, standing and walking, and hand function. The child may be ahead in one channel and behind in another channel. If some of the postural reactions and voluntary motion cannot be obtained in one channel, attempt them in another. For example:

(1) All techniques for head and shoulder control from 0–8 months in normal prone development may also be used with the child's head forward (face towards the ground when necessary), in sitting or standing with table support.

(2) All techniques for arm patterns can be carried out in any position, i.e. prone, supine, sitting, standing, kneeling upright.

(3) All techniques for pelvic stability may be carried out in prone developmental levels of weight bearing on both knees or one knee, or alternatively in standing leaning on the hands on a low box. In addition vertical pelvic fixation is trained in the standing positions and upright kneeling. Pelvic stability is trained in supine with *bridging* technique. Development of sitting does not contribute as much to pelvic control itself, but its contribution of head and trunk control is necessary for pelvic postural fixation on trunk in standing, kneeling and other positions.

93

(4) Supine development may be omitted if head lag is trained through side lying techniques, bringing hands to midline and grasp feet may also be trained in sitting development. Rise from sitting may be omitted if the child can roll over and rise from prone.

(5) Development of standing and walking seems to require training in the standing/walking positions and work in prone/supine contributes little except to correct abnormal joint postures. Sitting development builds up standing in that the head and trunk control developed in sitting will be used in standing.

For most children it is advisable to follow all the developmental channels given. With experience modifications will be obvious with each child and if not the above suggestions may be useful.

TECHNIQUES AND DEVELOPMENTAL 'SCATTER'

It is rare to have techniques from only one developmental stage for *all* the child's motor training. Use the assessment findings on each child and search for his particular problems at the different levels. Remember you will be helping the child:

(1) Establish motor abilities at one level with techniques to *augment* activity.
(2) Facilitate motor abilities at the next levels rather than the next level.

AGE OF CHILD AND TECHNIQUES

Select techniques according to developmental level and *not* according to chronological age. Use similar ideas on the treatment of deformity. Commence *functional training* of feeding, dressing, washing in babies, if they are at the appropriate developmental level (see Chapter 8).

It is unfortunate that some workers think treatment should be cut down in older children. Postural reactions and other motor controls may only mature much later and unless stimulated will remain dormant. Teachers and other personnel in the older child's life may be shown how to include motor development so that precious school time is not lost from the child's education. The child should not have to miss school in order to travel to physiotherapy departments elsewhere. Some children may have to have specific treatment sessions as special problems arise and before and after orthopaedic surgery. The physiotherapist at the child's school should work out ideas with the teacher to stimulate movement in the classroom, playground or in physical education. Extra effort also needs to be made to maintain contact with a child's parents.

Adjustment to the actual techniques according to the size of child is obvious. However, the same methods may be used for any age. Instructions to babies and children have to be given according to the level of understanding in the baby or child. (See also the sections in Chapter 4 on The development of attention and Cues for learning.)

ONSET AND TECHNIQUES

The planning of therapy and selection of techniques is not affected by the onset of the condition at birth, after birth or in later childhood. Response to therapy sometimes seems much quicker if the onset is sudden on a previously normal nervous system. However, ultimately spontaneous recovery and motor development in acquired brain lesions is as unpredictable as in babies born with apparent brain damage. Children with either congenital or acquired lesions warrant stimulation and corrective procedures so that the potential of any of their nervous systems is given every chance to reveal itself. Expectations of better results in children who have 'already known normal movements' may be more of a frustration than a help. It is not so much the memory and experience that matters but the amount of damage *and* the capacity of any particular damaged system to compensate for the abnormalities.

DIAGNOSIS AND TECHNIQUES

The techniques are not devised for particular diagnostic types but for motor problems of delay and abnormal performance. Different diagnostic types may have similar problems and even abnormal performances described may be seen in spastics, athetoids and ataxics as well as other forms of motor delay. This is especially so if abnormal performance is a compensation for delayed balance (postural mechanisms).

Techniques are given for both delay and abnormal performance. Some children may only have motor delay whilst others will have both delay and disorder. Diagnostic features of spasticity, rigidity (hypertonus), involuntary movement, hypotonicity are treated within the treatment suggestions in the motor developmental training throughout this chapter as well as in the treatment of deformity in Chapter 9, in the section on therapy and daily care. In Chapter 8, the section on motor function and feeding, dressing, toileting, washing, bathing, play and communication reviews positions which enable a child to master his symptoms. The section on Techniques for carrying the child correctly also minimizes the diagnostic symptoms.

APPLICATION OF TECHNIQUES

These should be carried out by qualified physiotherapists and occupational therapists and shown to anyone caring for the motor delayed and disabled child. Where techniques require a physiotherapist only, they have been labelled *physiotherapy suggestions*. Techniques which can be taught to others are labelled *treatment suggestions and daily care.* Selection of the appropriate technique for each child should be made by therapists and when necessary discussed with doctors and other team members.

Repertoire of techniques in this book cannot possibly include all those available. Firstly, not *all* individual problems could be included together with possible techniques. Secondly, it is difficult to describe techniques without demonstration and only those techniques which could be described have been included. Thirdly, those techniques which have been frequently used have been selected. There are many more.

Lack of response to any technique given in this book indicates the need to try others in this book or in other publications or preferably from clinical colleagues. Check that if the child scarcely responds to any technique, it is not due to:

(1) Inaccurate assessment of the child's level of development.
(2) Inadequate knowledge of the child's non-motor areas of function, i.e. understanding, perception, or other problems which interfere with carrying out movement.
(3) Lack of skill of the therapist with the particular technique.

MOTOR DEVELOPMENT AND CHILD'S DAILY LIFE

Although the techniques below concentrate on the motor problems, they are not isolated from other related areas of function. Wherever possible, motor activities have been interwoven with communication, sensation and perception. Such interactions are particularly obvious in the activities of the child's daily life. Chapter 8 summarizes the motor functions trained in this chapter in the contexts of feeding, dressing, playing, toileting, communication and perceptual experiences.

Although motor abilities in these contexts also train the motor function itself, and make it even more meaningful to the child, it is often too complex. Motor function needs to be isolated to some degree, to train the deficient motor apparatus. Similarly, perceptual problems or communication (speech and language) problems and special problems of, say, deafness and blindness should have structured, isolated sessions of training or therapy. Thus therapy has two main aspects:

(1) Specialized techniques for specific motor problems to initiate dormant motor activity, intensify correction and training of motor activity.
(2) Techniques to integrate motor function with related areas of function in the child's activities of daily living. Integration of movement with perception and cognition. This is for more effective motor learning.

Motor development and the child with severe visual impairment

Motor delay will occur because of the visual handicap in otherwise normal children. When cerebral palsy is also present the delay will be augmented. Intellectual disability may be present or only appear to be present as the child is limited by the multiple disabilities. The therapist should learn what influence the visual problems have on motor development as they do not only delay but also create unusual patterns and sequences of motor milestones. Abnormal movements or *blindisms* such as hand flapping, waving over light sources, eye poking, rocking and other bizarre patterns are seen in children, especially in some of the children referred late for training and parental advice. These will need special methods advised by psychologists.

The methods for motor developmental training in this book can be adapted for the visually handicapped child provided that the following factors are kept in mind.

HYPOTONIA, MOTOR DEVELOPMENT AND THE POSTURAL REACTIONS

As discussed throughout the book the postural reactions are undeveloped in children who are hypotonic (see the section on Postural mechanisms in Chapter 1 and the Hypotonicity sections in Chapters 3 and 9). Blind or sighted immobile children, delayed in motor development, may also be hypotonic. Floppyness or hypotonia is thus associated in blind babies with lack of movement (Jan *et al.* 1977; Sharby 1978). Assessment and development of the postural reactions in the visually handicapped baby and young child have been studied by the author. As vision is an important factor in detecting the vertical in the child's world and in appreciating any tilt of his world, it is not surprising that the blind baby's postural control is absent or poor. Blind babies prefer to lie safely on the ground and avoid the challenges of gravity. The development of the postural reactions is also the story of the development against gravity and changes in gravity. In effect it is the story of gross motor development. The visually handicapped child, with or without cerebral palsy, will need careful assessment and training of the postural reactions using auditory, tactile and increased proprioceptive and vestibular stimuli. As fears are common, the techniques should be adapted to build confidence and provide fun and a sense of adventure. Large balls, rolls and swings should only be used *after* confidence has been established and in relation to the levels of development of the postural reactions present or just commencing in the individual child.

Thus as for sighted babies with hypotonia, the development of the postural mechanisms will counteract the hypotonia and assist the development of motor abilities.

Poor posture such as rounded backs in sitting and standing, hyperextended knees and flat feet are common in sighted hypotonic children and particularly common in visually handicapped babies and children (Fig. 7.1). The specific delays in postural fixation, counterpoising, forward tilt and posterior saving reactions are often observed by the author to accompany the presence of round backs and shoulders. In addition, prone development which activates head and back extension is frequently poor. Vision provokes and monitors the postural mechanisms. Sugden (1992) reviews the studies on this aspect. It is the exciting object or person that a baby catches sight of that provokes him to look up. This then stimulates the head righting and postural fixation of the head. It is also the effort to understand the visual stimuli that further provokes exploratory movements and increasing postural control whilst exploring. Methods to develop the postural reactions or the motor abilities cannot be isolated from a child's total development (Zinkin 1979; Sykanda & Levitt 1982, Ch. 14; Levitt 1984; Sonksen *et al.* 1984).

TOTAL CHILD DEVELOPMENT AND MOTOR TRAINING

Mother—child relationships The shock and stress in the mother who does not even receive the *primal gaze* from her blind baby (Goldschmied 1975) as well as his unusual reactions to her feeding and cooing, must be understood by any therapist attempting to help. All motor developmental training must be designed to build up mother's and father's confidence in parenting their child. Many of the gross motor activities in play help enormously in creating bonds with the child. The techniques in this book should all be adapted to take place on mother's lap, close to her body and face so that her kisses, touch and stroking and talking to the baby not only help motor development but also body image, movement enjoyment by the baby and demonstrate to the baby love and security which

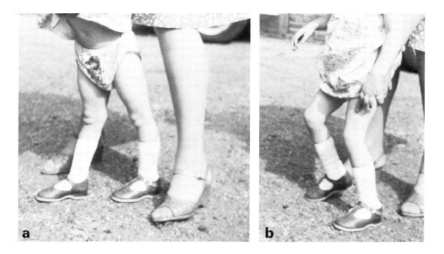

Fig. 7.1 Hyperextended knees (a) being corrected (b) by training pelvic control (postural fixation and counterpoising).

he needs so much. Clinging to mother in an unknown or puzzling world should be allowed for longer than in sighted babies and children. The weaning of the child with visual disability to a physiotherapist should be carefully done after mother–child bonding and confidence is established. Introducing more than one therapist or developmental worker may be disconcerting to the child and even the parents. Other disciplines must advise one therapist rather than all handle the child themselves. Family participation in helping and in enjoying the motor programme with a child who is visually impaired is planned by therapists. If mother is under stress it is important not to overload her with exercises, but rather use corrective movements and postures within the daily living activities of the child. Social workers and other counsellors work closely with therapists to help the family (see Chapter 5).

Motor function and the child's daily life (Chapter 8 in this book) is usually the priority in the developmental motor training programme for the child with visual disability, not only from the parent's viewpoint, but also from the child's viewpoint. The purpose of motor function must be conveyed to the blind baby and child (Fig. 7.2). If not, he could be trained in basic motor patterns but never use them. He cannot *see* their purpose!

The assessments of the child's developmental stages in feeding and other self care, play or sensory motor understanding and in exploration of his world must be obtained in order to introduce the corrective motor patterns appropriately. There are special stages and sequences for severe visual impairment (Reynell & Zinkin 1975; Kitzinger 1980).

Use of compensatory stimuli for motor development As vision is not available, it seems obvious to use auditory and tactile stimuli to provoke motor development. However, it is vision which normally teaches the baby what makes sounds, where they come from in direction and in distance, how humans communicate and the association of sounds with situations such as meal times, bath times and so on. Therefore, first train the baby what sounds mean before they can really motivate him to move. Also use existing movements to confirm what sounds mean.

Auditory development is followed as observed in the normal child (Sheridan 1975) but with special adaptations for the visual impairment (Sonksen 1979). First, the baby is trained to listen, then to turn to sound and after that to reach for sound. He will first localize the source of sound near his ears horizontally and then above and below him. He must be helped kinaesthetically to search for the sound *kept stationary* near him. Developmentally this will be at ear level, horizontally, above, below and then behind the child. The child will *only* achieve reach for sound when his conceptual development includes *the permanence of objects* and their sounds. It is at about these stages that reach and move towards a sound will only be worth using to stimulate roll over, creeping, crawling

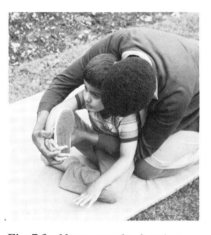

Fig. 7.2 Movements for dressing.

or bottom shuffling. Until the permanence of objects is conceptualized, help the child locate sound and move towards it by providing tactile and kinaesthetic stimuli.

Similarly the appreciation of tactile stimuli, localizing and searching for them, has to be developed. Linking tactile with sound stimuli must be carried out. Encouraging the child to create sound himself should be included as he bangs a mobile, rattle, tambourine or a surface with hands or feet. The motor programme cannot be planned without these aspects which are devised by teachers, psychologists and developmental paediatricians together with the therapist.

Mother's voice and her touch rather than the therapist's will be more successful in the early stages. Vibration, smell, taste and air currents can be introduced. Link sound, touch, proprioception and vestibular stimuli. All these aspects are associated with the child's conceptual development (Sonksen *et al.* 1984).

Body image development Poor body image is related to poor motor experiences and not seeing body parts static or moving. The tactile stimuli are used to develop the body image. However, it is the mother's and the baby's hands that should do the touching first. Hands of the baby are notoriously slow to move and explore because of many reasons, not least of which is the absence of *hand regard*. Help the baby bring his hands together in midline, *pat-a-cake* hand to hand, touch hand to mouth, hand to body and hand to feet (see Fig. 7.3). Later use as many other

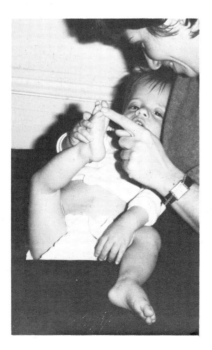

Fig. 7.3 Body image development.

stimuli to his body such as rubbing with towels, soap, creams and powder at bath time. Use vibrating toys, bells, and playthings placed for him to find on his tummy, legs and similar ideas. The sections on Stages of hand function development in this chapter and motor function and perception in Chapter 8 offer ideas for the sighted child in this book. For the child without sight these stimuli offered in play activities should be emphasized and also *presented more slowly* and stage by stage. Do not bombard the baby with too many stimuli at once. Confusion or fear could be aroused if stimuli are not sensitively given. Thus, carefully introduce different surfaces for the child to roll on, creep, crawl, and walk on with bare feet.

Always give the child time to experience tactile and auditory stimuli and let him reach and find out about them himself whenever possible. He feels his own body movements and how he actively produced them. If he does not move himself, parents must move him, changing positions for him. He should feel his mother move about by being slung close to her body in a baby pack.

Proprioceptive and vestibular function These aspects are also part of total child development. They are compensatory stimuli for visual handicap and also develop body image. All the postural reactions are dependent on these stimuli in a developmental context discussed in this book. Touch, pressure and resistance can be correctly given to stimulate movement giving clues as to direction and degree of muscle action. However, as with all therapy methods, observe whether the child understands and is not confused by what is expected of him. Do not use therapy techniques with handling, pressures, or other proprioceptive stimuli from behind him as he may well lean back or use his extensor thrusts to reach the stimuli or the familiar voice behind him! Body image training is also stimulation of proprioception and vestibular input for the visually impaired child.

Visual development Not all blind babies are totally blind. Even reaction to light only, can be used and perhaps developed to the child's full if limited capacities. An assessment of the developmental *use* of residual vision is given by the developmental paediatrician and guides the therapist in her motor plan for the individual child. The physiotherapist should be told how large an object can be seen by the child, how far away, whether it can be seen if stationery or moving and which visual fields are present. Equality of vision in each eye and the acuity as well as any special visual defects which may affect handling the child and motor development should also be known. Vision for exploration and for learning is assessed by the developmental paediatrician. Development of visual potential is easily integrated with the methods for head control, hand function and all balance and locomotor activities discussed in this book. Once again, relate the appropriate level of visual ability with the child's motor programme. Also one may have to accept unusual head position and other patterns which make it possible for the child to use residual vision.

Language development   It is important to talk and clearly label the body parts used, the motor activity and generally encourage the child's language development. Delay is *normal* for a child who cannot yet understand the meaning of sounds, words and conversation as he cannot see what they mean, cannot see gestures and cannot link the stimuli from the external world. Psychologists and teachers work closely with the therapists to plan the language and speech programme.

Communication is also fostered through motor actions, touch and body language relevant to the visually handicapped child. Psychologists and speech therapists will advise on these aspects.

Motor developmental sequences   The development of hand function is obviously the most important area for the child whose hands are his eyes on the world. The hand function chapter in this book should be adapted to use compensatory tactile, auditory and proprioceptive stimuli before motor actions can be expected to follow the normal rate of development. Do not force objects into the child's hand but train him to search for the nearby rattle, to orientate his hand to take it and to develop a variety of searching actions or finger moulding and feeling actions. Bilateral hand function will take more work than with the sighted child. Encourage both hands together in midline, holding and especially exploring both sides of a cup, bowl, ball or toy and transfer of toys. Train losing the toy and finding it and taking it apart, constructing it again. Also train crude and fine voluntary release. All these actions must link with the concept of object permanence and other intellectual development of the child. Remember that index finger pointing and associated index/first finger grasp is very much a visual skill and will be delayed. Offer toys and food to promote finger actions as mentioned in the chapters on hand function, motor function and play, feeding and other self care activities.

Prone development is not popular with the visually handicapped baby as there is no interest there, sounds cannot be heard as easily and he may be far removed from family and especially mother. There are no visual lures to provoke him to look up and progress to creeping and crawling. It is often noted that crawling is not used by blind children and that they prefer shuffling on their bottoms and then walking. It is possible to train prone development on mother's lap, on a soft cushion with attractive noises especially mother's voice and her stroking her child's back. The advantages are increased head and back muscle strength due to head and back extension and coming up on hands, hands and knees and development of an additional exploratory skill of crawling through space and of additional body image experiences for the child. The round backs and shoulders may be helped by stronger back extensors but additional postural training in sitting and counterpoising of the arms when reaching up for toys or mother's face helps more.

Crawling is not of course essential for the acquisition of walking, as bottom shufflers demonstrate. It is the crawling, rolling or movement across space and much learning experiences of space and especially that the floor is continuous that teaches the child to be less afraid and to walk alone. Walkers with wheels all around the child should be avoided as he will not develop his own postural and locomotive reactions. The child often sits or leans onto these walkers, stepping his legs but not learning to take weight through his legs and so learn to walk. Baby bouncers and rocking chairs are also of potential danger if unsupervised. Withdrawal into a rocking world can be engendered and bouncing may provoke abnormal leg patterns, excessive toe-walking (*blindism*) and spasticity and athetosis. Short supervised sessions in any equipment do often produce more desirable results, especially if mother–child interaction is included.

Blind babies develop postures slightly later or within the ranges of sighted developmental levels (Fraiberg 1977). However, there is more of a delay of moving into, or out of or forward from these postures. Thus, this book on developmental levels should be used as guidelines and not as rigid rules for developmental ages nor strict sequences for the visually handicapped. The postural reactions of fixation, counterpoising, tilt and saving (protective) reactions and the methods given are in a logical sequence for therapy, but delays and modifications will be required according to the particular vision and hearing development, emotional and social situations and the amount of developmental intervention given. Rising reactions will require extra care as all workers in this field demonstrate how much visual lures promote posture changes. All other motor developmental training from 0 to 5 years presented in this book should be continued to avoid the frequently occurring clumsiness in the visually handicapped. Co-ordination exercises, balance tasks, music and movement, dance, games and physical education are of great value to the children with visual disabilities. The older child will also be receiving mobility training from those employed for this work by the Royal National Institute for the Blind. Teachers of the blind will integrate their work on this and other aspects with the therapists, as there is a need to create a whole programme for each child and family.

PRONE DEVELOPMENT

The following main features should be developed:

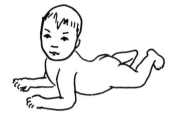

Fig. 7.4a Postural fixation of head and shoulder girdle (on forearms).

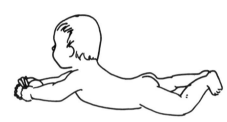

Fig. 7.4b Postural fixation of head and shoulder girdle.

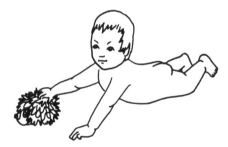

Fig. 7.4c Postural fixation and counterpoising arm reach.

Postural fixation of the head (Fig. 7.4a–d) when lying prone (0–3 months), on forearms (3 months), on hands and on hands and knees (6 months), during crawling, half-kneeling hand support (9–11 months) or in the *bear walk* (12 months) in normal developmental levels.

Postural fixation of the shoulder girdle (Fig. 7.4b–d) when taking weight on forearms (3 months), on hands (6 months), on hands and knees and arms stretched forward along the ground to hold a toy at 5–6 months also include postural fixation. Pivot prone or the *Landau type* of posture with arms held extended and in the air also provokes postural fixation (8–10 months). Maintenance of half-kneeling lean on hands or upright kneeling lean on hands or grasp a support are other normal developmental motor activities around 9–12 months which stimulate shoulder girdle fixation.

Counterpoising of the head takes place in activities which include head turn and head movements whilst holding the head up against gravity.

Counterpoising the arm movements at about 5 months normal level when in prone lean on one forearm reach with the other or 7 months lean on hand reach with the other (Fig. 7.4c). Reach in all directions increases counterpoising ability as well as other features of motor ability.

Postural fixation of the pelvis (Fig. 7.4d) on knees with hips at right angles (4 months), on elbows and knees and on hands and knees (4–6

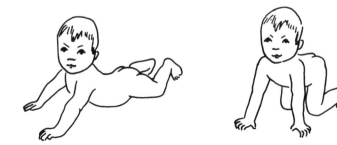

Fig. 7.4d Postural fixation on hands and on hands and knees.

months), on one knee with the other foot flat as in half-kneeling and upright kneeling with support (9–12 months) in normal motor levels.

Counterpoising movement of one leg takes place on knees with upper trunk and arms supported (5–6 months), on hands and knees (6–8 months) together with counterpoising of arm motion in crawling (9–11 months), in bear walk (12 months). Stand lean on hands on low table, carry out leg patterns in each leg also trains counterpoising in normal developmental levels (see Development of standing at 9–12 months normal developmental stages in this chapter).

Rising from prone (Fig. 7.5) head (0–3 months), on to forearms (3 months), on to knees (4 months), on to forearms and knees (5–6 months), on to hands and knees (6–7 months), to half-kneeling hand support (9–12 months), prone to standing without support (12–18 months). Change from and to prone, sitting, squatting, crawling positions (10 months) and other positions with further motor development.

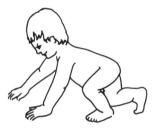

Fig. 7.5 Rising from prone.

Tilt reactions in prone (Fig. 7.6) Reactions seen on tilting the surface on which the child lies at about 6 months; on hands and knees at about 9–12 months.

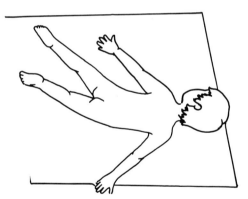

Fig. 7.6 Tilt reaction in prone.

Saving from falling reactions (Fig. 7.7) in the arms at 5–7 months downward-and-forward parachute, and propping. Arm and leg reactions accompany the tilt reactions in prone, especially if the trunk reaction is particularly poor. Other saving reactions are described in the sitting development. Arm saving sideways and forward can also be seen in prone, on hands and knees, if the child is suddenly pushed sideways or forward from a heel-sitting position, or when on hands and knees on a rocking board. Leg reactions also occur on pushing the child over sideways, forward, or backward when he is on hands and knees.

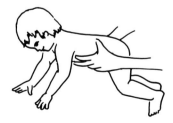

Fig. 7.7 Saving reactions in the arms.

Stages in prone development (Figs 7.8–7.22)

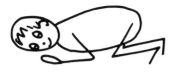

Fig. 7.8 Flexion posture decreases. Head turn (*0–3 months*)

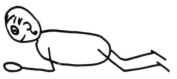

Fig. 7.9 Head raise and hold (*0–3 months*).

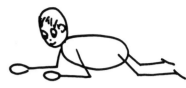

Fig. 7.10 Head raise, weight on forearms (*0–3 months*).

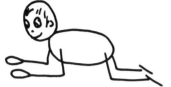

Fig. 7.11 On forearms and/or weight bearing on knees (*3–6 months*).

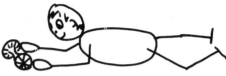

Fig. 7.12 Stretch forward to reach; stretch legs. Lean on one forearm and reach with the other arm (*3–6 months*).

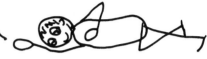

Fig. 7.13 Roll from prone to supine (*3–6 months*).

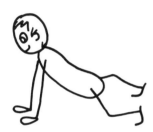

Fig. 7.14 Weight bearing on hands (*6–9 months*).

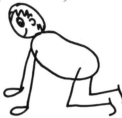

Fig. 7.15 Weight bearing on hands and knees (*6–9 months*).

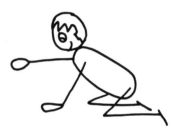

Fig. 7.16 Lean on one hand reach with the other (*7 months*).

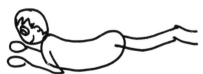

Fig. 7.17 Extend head, shoulders, hips–pivot prone position (*8 months*).

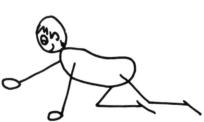

Fig. 7.18 Hands and knees, lift arm, leg or both (*8 months*).

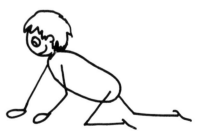

Fig. 7.19 Crawling. Rise into crawl position. (*9 months*).

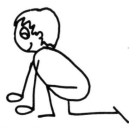

Fig. 7.20 Half-kneeling lean on hands. (*11 months*).

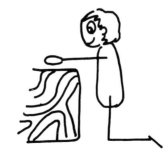

Fig. 7.21 Kneeling supported (*11 months*).

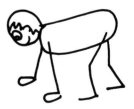

Fig. 7.22 Bear-walk (elephant walk) on hands and feet (*12 months*).

Stages in prone development

0–3 Months normal developmental level

SOME COMMON PROBLEMS

Dislike of prone position   This may be due to early breathing difficulties, inability to turn the head and free the nose, inability to lift the head up, excessive flexion creating discomfort in prone or even lack of opportunity given to lie on his stomach. Later a dislike of prone may be due to the child's inability to use his hands in prone.

Delayed development of head control, rising up on forearms, taking weight on forearms.

Abnormal performance (Fig. 7.23), e.g. asymmetrical head raise, rising on one forearm only, asymmetrical stabilization on elbows, excessive flexion of either of the arms (often caught under the child's body) or flexion of the trunk or legs, or all of them. The head may overextend when raised. There may be more flexion-adduction in one leg than the other as the hips lift off the surface into flexion. One leg may flex and abduct into a forward creeping pattern with hips flexed off the surface or flat. This asymmetry of flexion is often greater in spastic diplegia than in quadri-

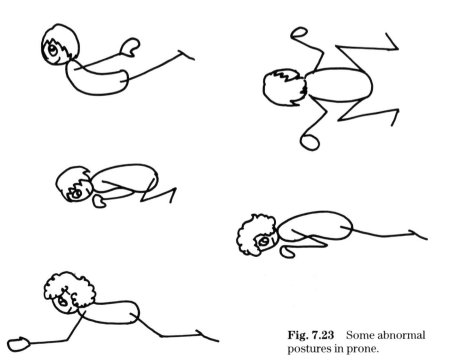

Fig. 7.23   Some abnormal postures in prone.

plegia. Athetoid quadriplegia and floppy babies tend to flex and abduct both legs outwards into the *frog position*. Hemiplegic children begin to creep and flex the good side whilst the hemiplegic side goes into extension – internal rotation. This is seen especially when the child raises his head and turns to the good side. Independent head raising in the other cerebral palsied children is usually associated with flexion in the arms but extension of the back and especially of the legs into adduction-internal rotation. In normal babies the leg extension (especially at the next developmental level) is associated with abduction and external rotation.

Reflex reactions in prone   Flexor reaction to prone: arm flexor reaction: Galant's response, neck righting not beginning to diminish. Appearance of head righting may be delayed.

TREATMENT SUGGESTIONS AND DAILY CARE

Acceptance of prone position   Accustom the child to prone by placing him slowly on his stomach and on soft surfaces, such as sponge rubber, inflatable mattress, in warm water, over large rubber beach ball, over your lap (adding a cushion if your knees are bony!). Gently bring his bent arms away from his chest and place them over an edge or curved surface, rock and sway a baby held in prone suspension. The child's face should be over the edge of the surface with the nose free. Training should be given to help him turn his head to the side, if he cannot do this (see below).

The child may also be suspended in a blanket or hammock and gently rolled from side lying into prone lying and back until he accepts that last roll into prone lying. His nose should be over the edge of the blanket as he rolls over.

Note   Some children continue to strongly refuse to go prone and should not be forced to do so. Some of these are like normal children who are *rollers* or *bottom shufflers* and a few others who do not use prone development in their motor behaviour (Robson 1970).

Head control   Train these aspects of head control:

- Raising the head (righting).
- Holding the head steady (postural fixation).
- Turning the head from side to side (counterpoising and movement).

(1)   Place the child in prone across a sponge rubber roll, a beach ball, a wedge, pile of pillows or across your lap. Then elevate his arms and gently stretch them symmetrically across the surface or over the edge of the surface. Stiff arms may first have to be grasped near the

shoulder joints and turned outwards as they are extended forwards over the edge of the apparatus or on the ball. If he reaches out actively, his head often raises as well. The child's legs may be abnormally bent or stiffly extended, turned in and held together, before or only during head raising. In such cases turn them out and keep his legs apart *while* he is obtaining head control (Fig. 7.24).

Rock the child forward and backwards over the edge of the roll/ball or inflatable mattress. Rhythmically tap under the child's chin to give momentum to lift the head. Tapping the child's forehead also helps if he does not like having his face touched. Hold the child's shoulders on both sides symmetrically.

(2) Bring his shoulders back and inwards towards his spine – this provokes him to head raise. If the child persists in abnormal turning of his head to one side, then extend the shoulder girdle on the opposite side to provoke head turn and raise to that side (Fig. 7.25).

(3) With the child's head over the edge present him with interesting visual and auditory stimuli, slightly above him and also in front of

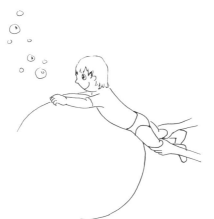

Fig. 7.24

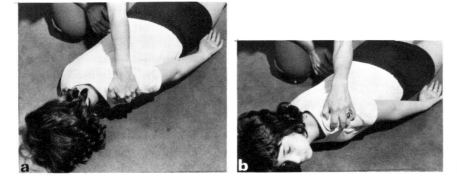

Fig. 7.25

Fig. 7.29a Measurements for wedge for prone lying, arms over edge 'A'. A, Measurement from axilla to wrist. B, Measurement from axilla to 2 in (50 mm) above ankle, C, Length to top of foot.

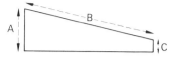

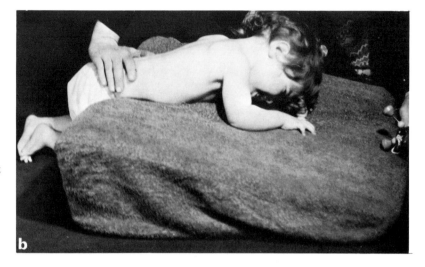

Fig. 7.29b Use wedge for weight bearing on knees or reversed for weight bearing on elbows or on hands, stimulation of head raise, and use of hands on the floor. Straps may be needed to hold the child on the wedge.

gently push his weight over and hold him on to the weaker weight-bearing side. As soon as possible remove your support and do not hold him during play. Do this also during feeding, washing and other activities in sitting position.

(2) When the child is in prone lying over a roll, pillows or wedge, press down firmly through his head in line with his neck (*chin in and long neck*) or down through the top of his shoulders increasing his weight bearing on to his elbows (see Figs 7.101, 7.102).

(3) Hold baby with his full weight through his elbows or on one elbow. Slightly shift his weight, first on to one elbow and then on to the other elbow. An older child can do this if you hold his legs up in the air while he takes weight on to his forearms. Hold spastic legs apart, turned outward and with straight hips and knees.

Note Always try removing any supports given by your hands or equipment to check whether the child can lift his head or take weight on forearms on his own momentarily and with practice reliably. Train a *long neck* with chin held in as well as head extension.

PHYSIOTHERAPY SUGGESTIONS

Abnormal postures Excessive flexion and other abnormal postures are corrected by the stimulation of head raise symmetrically, head turn to non-preferred side, weight bearing on forearms at right-angles to chest, stretching child out symmetrically over rolls, wedges, mother's lap and by active extension movements and the active creeping patterns. General corrective positioning on special wedges and knee or elbow gaiters may be needed.

(1) *Facilitate symmetrical head raising* by either holding both the child's shoulders in rotation-extension or both arms elevated, abducted-external rotation behind the plane of his head or by asking him to push his elevated arms back against your hands pressing against his upper arms and straight elbows, or by use of the creeping arm pattern carried out in the plane behind the child's head. Try to activate the chin in and long neck posture.

(2) *Facilitate head raise and turn* as in Fig. 7.25 or by lifting the elevated arm on one side back and behind the child's head to provoke the creeping pattern (Fig. 7.30a).

Creeping patterns It is difficult to describe these patterns without

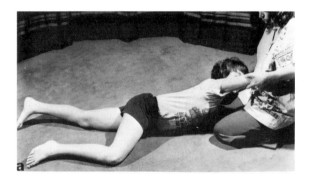

Fig. 7.30

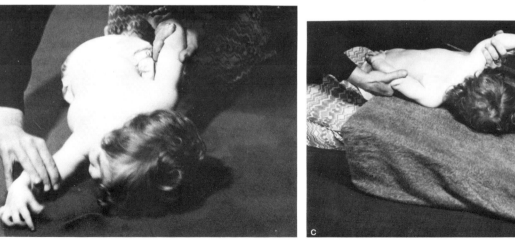

demonstration. Some aspects will be described as these techniques are particularly helpful.

The *face arm* is elevated into shoulder abduction-external rotation (Fig. 7.30b). The *occiput arm* is brought down into shoulder extension-adduction internal rotation (Fig. 7.30c). The child may lie flat on the surface or over the edge of a roll, small pillow or wedge.

(1)   Assisted active changing of the arms so that the opposite arm is elevated whilst the face arm moves down. These arm actions facilitate head raise and turn, back extension and leg creeping movements.

(2)   Use of stretch-rotation and appropriate resistance activates the creeping movements.

(3)   The child may continue active creeping on his own and so acquire one form of locomotion beginning at this level of development.

(4)   If the elevated *face arm* is held stationary by your hand or a firm padded object, you can concentrate on facilitating the creeping forward action of the *occiput arm* against your manual or just thumb resistance. If the child understands, ask him to pull his arm forward and above his head. An automatic rising reaction on to the forearm of the face arm occurs. In some babies and severely affected older children, the stretch of the occiput arm especially with extension-rotation of the shoulder girdle on that side, provokes the same automatic rise on to the forearm of the face arm. As the child rises, he also raises and turns his head.

(5)   Facilitation of leg creeping involves single leg flexion-abduction-external rotation, preferably with pelvic rotation backward. The other leg is held in extension-adduction-*external* rotation. Legs should be held at the thigh and knee using stretch-rotation and resistance according to the child's reaction. (See also Fig. 7.30a.)

(6)   Like arm creeping, the facilitation of the leg motion counteracts abnormal postures of the legs, trunk flexion and arm flexion against chest (arm flexor reaction; reaction to prone).

Active leg creeping may facilitate active automatic arm creeping actions. For example, hold one of the child's legs at the thigh and knee and stretch it into extension-adduction external rotation. A quick stretch into this pattern provokes a *recoil* towards flexion-abduction-external rotation which is the forward creeping motion of the leg. If the child understands, ask him to bend his hip and knee up and out against your hand. Offer him enough resistance to augment his movement.

As the leg creeps forward and especially if it is guided into full external rotation with pelvic rotation backwards, there is an automatic arm creeping forward, usually on the same side or on the contralateral (opposite) side. This creeping technique is useful for activation of more affected arms or arm as in hemiplegic babies or mentally impaired severely affected children.

(7) Rising reactions may be provoked if the flexion-abduction-externally rotated leg is held fixed manually or by a padded box. The other leg is provoked into flexion-abduction-external rotation as above. The effect may be rising on to the forearms, the hands or the knee on the fixed or stationary side. Rising on to knees is more likely in children in the developmental level of 4–6 months. (See Fig. 7.34 at the next level of development.)

There are many possibilities for rising reactions and other stabilising and movement reactions with Vojta's creeping techniques and my own modifications. However, they have to be demonstrated and supervision given by specialised physiotherapists.

Modified creeping over mother's lap or down a slippery wedge/incline is enjoyed by children.

Facilitate rising on to both forearms or later hands at the same time. Hold the child's head by spanning his occiput between his ears. Ask him to raise his head up against your manual pressure. This pressure and sometimes manual resistance facilitates rising on to his forearms or hands, and, shows him what to do.

Augment head holding, and forearm support by resistance to head hold, as well as head raise. Encourage child to pull his chin inwards getting *a long neck*. Also give manual resistance to front, side, back of shoulders, as child is told to 'stay there' or 'don't let me push you down' or simply 'hold it'.

Note Use of resistance is recommended for athetoids and ataxics and weak developmentally disabled children. In spastic children resistance should be controlled so that there is no abnormal overflow such as extensor spasms or flexor spasms.

4–6 Months normal developmental level

COMMON PROBLEMS

Delay in acquisition of rising on knees, rising on to hands with straight elbows, weight bearing on knees, knees and forearms and on one forearm, reaching for objects, inability to lie prone with both or one of the arms stretched and reaching overhead, unable to roll over to supine, or unable to creep on abdomen, on elbows or with various creeping movements of both arms and legs.

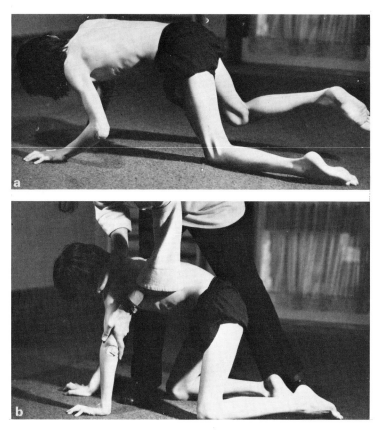

Fig. 7.33

(1) Weight bearing on one forearm, reach with the other. Weight bear and shift from forearm to forearm. Encourage reach with one arm on floor, then above his head and in different positions. Do this during daily activities.

(2) With the child bearing weight on both forearms give him toys in each hand to grasp and play with. Let him grasp the ends of a bicycle pump, concertina, plastic bottle, transparent cylinder with coloured water or marbles inside, grasp two balls or blocks to bang together or push a ball from hand to hand. Toys should move or make a noise if touched, patted, pressed or grasped. Remove the wedge and hold the child on one of his forearms while he actively uses the other arm in play. Whenever possible remove adult support altogether (see the section on Development of hand function in this chapter).

(3) Child in prone lying on forearms on thick soft sponge, inflatable mattress, water bed, trampoline, press the surface down on each side so that the child tips on to his elbow. Do this to a song or rhythm.

(4)   Child may weight shift from one forearm to the other forearm in order to creep along the floor. As the child creeps on his abdomen with weight shift on the forearms it is best if the legs are held up, turned out and apart in cases where the legs stiffen into abnormal positions with thighs pressed together or turned in during this activity of creeping or *walking on the elbows* or *wheelbarrow on forearms*. You can also place the child on a low platform or low wedge on wheels with the legs held in abduction with abduction pants or a pommel. The child should be shown how to use his elbow walking *backwards*. If he is on a bed and wishes to get off he could then move himself backwards so that his legs come off the edge of the bed, his feet take the weight and he can stand up leaning on elbows.

Note   Do *not* use this activity in those cases where there is a tendency to tight elbow flexion and shoulder hunching but rather practise weight bearing on one elbow stretching out for toys with the other arm and also stretching both arms well forward to toy or to push a big ball away.

Arms stretched overhead and forward: arm saving reactions in prone: propping reactions

(1)   Encourage the child to reach forward and overhead for toys, to push away a ball, balloon or toy on wheels. Older children can walk their hands up a wall or wall bars as far as possible (Fig. 9.1). Use a small bolster or wedge to help him stretch his arms out *and* up towards toys on a box or suspended above him.
(2)   Place the child over a beach ball or large roll with his arms over the top. Tip the ball forward and encourage him to reach for the ground to save himself from falling. Encourage him to prop himself on his hands by placing his hands on the ground, to *stand on his hands* whilst you hold his body safely on the ball. You can hold a young child and tip him upside down near a surface, e.g. a table, and encourage him to put his arms out to save himself and then to take weight on them (Fig. 7.48).
(3)   Place the child on his abdomen on a large cushion with his arms stretched forward, and help him to go down a slide head first. Also tip a horizontal stationary cushion downwards to provoke arm saving reaction.

Note   The therapist needs to check whether positions of arms and legs are correct during all the activities above, for example:

●   Shoulders and hips at right angles in weight bearing positions.
●   Knees pointed outwards without a *frogging* position.
●   Hips and knees straight, apart, and if possible turned outwards.

- Shoulders and arms turned out rather than inward.
- Hands open and palms down if weight bearing.

It is important to recognize that *all the training* of weight bearing on elbows, one elbow, hands may be done in *sitting* or *standing* leaning forward down on to a low table or box. This reinforces the prone development *or* if prone is occasionally not indicated for a particular child, these activities can and need to be trained in these other positions.

Rolling from prone to supine See physiotherapy suggestions for rolling and roll-and-rise in the section on supine development.

PHYSIOTHERAPY SUGGESTIONS

Facilitate rising for assumption of four-point position (forearms and knee position).

(1) Fix one of the child's legs in creeping position with a box or manually (Fig. 7.34). Press down through his buttocks. You may hold his other leg above or below the knee and stretch it into extension – adduction – external rotation provoking a creeping movement forward. If the child understands he should be instructed to *bend* his hip and knee. If this movement is fully resisted by the therapist no movement occurs but instead the child will *right* or rise up on his other knee, or on to his arms. Note the automatic creeping forward of this baby's right arm.
(2) Hold the child under his upper arms. Rotate his arms and his trunk to one side to facilitate creeping forward of one leg. Rotate him to the other side so that he rises up on to both knees.

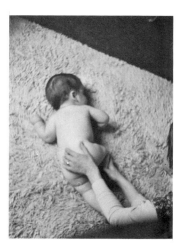

Fig. 7.34

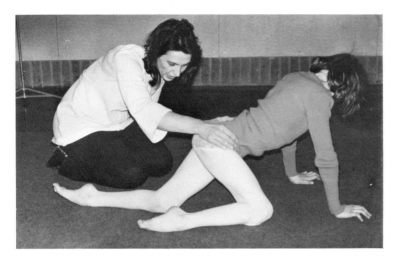

Fig. 7.35

(3) When the child is actively able to commence or even complete rising up on to knees and forearms, but is weak, then resistance is used to reinforce his efforts. Apply manual resistance at the pelvis in a diagonal direction (Fig. 7.35).

See roll-and-rise (Fig. 7.68).

Facilitate rising on to hands by using the same techniques as rising on to elbows at 4–6 months level above, but this time expecting child to rise all the way on to hands (6–9 months).

Augment holding on hands and knees
(1) The child attempts to maintain this position as the therapist slowly pushes him:
  • laterally at each hip or each shoulder
  • anteroposteriorly at hip or shoulders
  • at opposite shoulder and hip
  • at shoulder and hip on the same side.
(2) Resistance to head movements and to shoulders *stay there* (see on forearms, above). Similarly use resistance for hips when child is on knees with chest and arms supported by roll or stool.

6–9 Months normal developmental level

COMMON PROBLEMS

Delay in weight bearing on hands and knees, in lifting one or two limbs, weight bearing on one hand and reaching for objects, crawling on hands or on knees, pivot position and absence of rising from prone to hands and knees.

Abnormal performance of motor abilities, over-flexed hips, knees or feet, internally rotated legs or arms, lack of reciprocation in crawling, *bunny hopping* both knees forward in heel sitting, asymmetrical weight bearing. Prone *mermaid crawl* or *commando crawl* by pulling forward on his flexed arms with his legs stiffly extended, adducted and internally rotated. The hands may clench with each *pull* forward and often the legs adduct strongly with this pull.

Lack of postural fixation of the pelvis and hips creates creeping on the abdomen and masks the child's ability to take weight on hands at 6 months level of the development of crawling on all fours.

Absence of reactions expected at 6–9 months level in prone, absence of Landau, saving reactions in arms, tilting reactions in prone. Persistence of any early reactions, see 0–3 months level.

TREATMENT SUGGESTIONS AND DAILY CARE

See Figs 7.32 and 7.33 and add the following.

Weight bearing on one hand, reach for a toy and on hands and knees lift one arm or leg or both Place the child on hands or on hands and knees over rolls or your arm and when possible let him balance on his own:

(1) Lift individual limbs whilst he maintains balance to a song or counts.
(2) While child takes weight on his hands or hands and knees, encourage him to stroke different textures on the ground, e.g. carpets, linoleum, cool and warm surfaces, scratchy and smooth surfaces.
(3) While balancing on hands and knees he might scrub the floor or soap the linoleum, reach for a dangling toy, roll balls, move small toys on wheels, dig into the sandpit with one hand or a spade, on the grass he could pick flowers, handfuls of grass and so on. He can stretch a leg to kick tinkling toy bells, or touch a person.

Crawling This can be trained with the child:

(1) Suspended in a blanket. Hold each end of the blanket and tip the child in it so that his weight is taken more on one side releasing the other side for a 'step' forward.
(2) On a crawler. Hold the child's knees and point them outwards. Move one knee in front of the other. Tip the child on to the weight bearing knee as you guide the moving knee.

Note   It is important to avoid the use of crawlers and the training of crawling in children who have tight hip and knee flexors. In these cases use a wedge on wheels or platform on wheels with towels rolled under the child's chest so that his elbows are straight and his arms reach for the floor. The child crawls on his hands whilst his legs are held extended on the platform. See also wheelbarrow on forearms and do the same but as *wheelbarrow on hands*. In cases of severe knee and elbow flexion, splintage of these joints should be used as the child gets about on his platform on wheels.

Rolling   Encourage rolling on grass down a slight incline, on sponge rubber, on an inflatable mattress or down a mound (see Treatment suggestions and daily care for rolling and rising).

PHYSIOTHERAPY SUGGESTIONS

Flexion or lack of postural fixation of head, shoulder girdle and hips in extension or flexion positions may be treated with techniques above or with pivot prone (Fig. 7.36). Pivot prone or Landau position provoked by head raise:

- This can also be carried out on a large ball, roll.
- Also elevate-abduct-externally rotate arms behind plane of head.
- Abduct-extend and externally rotate legs in this child when she is on a roll.
- Older children may abduct-externally rotate shoulders in postural fixation by pulling against weights over pulleys opposite them.

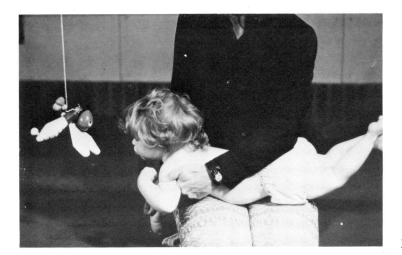

Fig. 7.36

Abdomen on low stool which supports the child at the chest and abdomen but allows extension in head and limbs is used.

Note The extension in pivot prone is not enough for standing. Postural fixation of the head, trunk and hips in the vertical must be trained (see the section on Development of standing and walking).

Counterpoising exercises Child maintains balance on hands and knees and carries out arm or leg patterns to achieve counterpoising (Fig. 7.37).

Leg pattern Ask the child to bend one knee up to the ceiling; manually resist his knee flexion forward and outward. Then reverse to hip and knee extension with adduction and external rotation (Figs 7.38–7.40). Resistance given to leg pattern will also increase stabilization at the shoulder girdle and opposite hip.

Arm pattern Use creeping pattern of child's arm from extension-adduction-internal rotation behind his back, facilitated to elevation-abduction-external rotation as described at the earlier levels (Fig. 7.30). Other arm patterns are arm flexion adduction across chest, change to abduction-extension-external rotation with trunk rotation backwards. As the child moves his one arm against resistance, he increases weight bearing or stabilization on the other three points. If he is on his hands only, abdomen on the floor, shoulder stabilization and counterpoising are stimulated, as follows: he balances on the one hand as single arm pattern of movement is carried out actively or against correctly given resistance.

(1) Continue pivoting in flexed children as above (Fig. 7.36).
(2) Continue rising on to hands *and* knees as above or roll-and-rise (see Fig. 7.68a and b in Supine development).

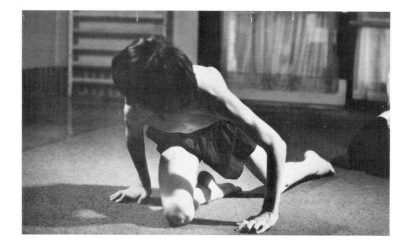

Fig. 7.37 Instability of pelvic and shoulder girdles and counterpoising.

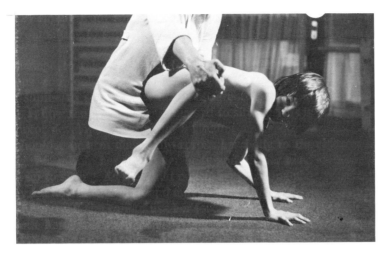

Fig. 7.38   Counterpoising exercises.

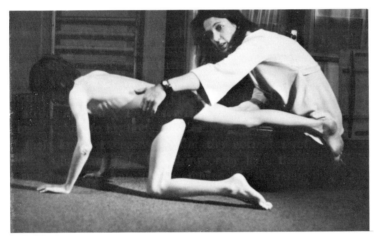

Fig. 7.39   Counterpoising exercises.

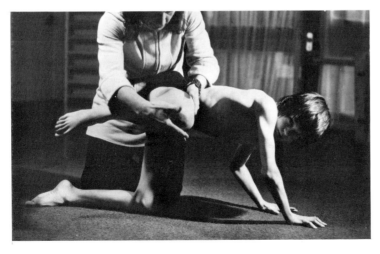

Fig. 7.40   Positions of therapist's hands. Child's leg flexion against hand on thigh or pull against hand on tibia. Leg extension against hand on tibia.

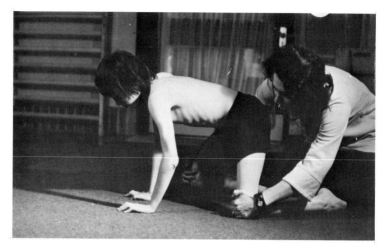

Fig. 7.41 Crawling against manual resistance of therapist – guidance or resistance of knee into external rotation avoids adduction and offers a wider base for balance.

(3) Child crawls against resistance given to his knees. Grasp his knees and guide them outward as you resist each step forward (Fig. 7.41).

(4) Augment holding on hands and knees (as above), especially the hips in bunny hoppers. Suggestions to discourage bunny hopping are given below.

Items 3 and 4 overlap into the next stage of development.

9–12 Months normal developmental level

COMMON PROBLEMS

Delay in easy reciprocal crawling, maintaining half-kneeling position hands on ground, on hands and feet and other more advanced postures. Absence of rising from hands and knees to standing holding a support and inability to change from prone to sitting, prone to squatting, prone to supported half-kneeling; grasping support or hands on floor and other changes of posture.

Abnormal performance Spastic adduction-internal rotation of hips in crawling, in half-kneeling and weight bearing on hands and feet. If the child can *bear walk* on hands and feet, he has his heels off the ground and/or excessive flexion of the knees with hips internally rotated and adducted.

Absence of reflex reactions expected at 9–12 months in prone, Landau, saving reaction in arms fully developed. Persistence of remnants of earlier reflex reactions, see previous levels.

TREATMENT SUGGESTIONS AND DAILY CARE

Half-kneeling Sit the child on the side of your lap when you sit on the ground. Bring his outside knee on to the floor, he is then kneeling on one knee, hold the other knee forward and outward. Remove your lap and place his hands on the floor for support. Encourage him to play in this position by moving a car or rolling a ball under the *bridge* of his knee, round his foot, or spend time in tying his boot laces, count his toes, paint his toe nails and so on. Later, he should grasp horizontal bars, at various levels, place his hands flat on the wall, low tables or your flat hands. Half-kneeling position should be maintained with the front knee pointing outward. Hold his knee out with his foot pointing out and placed out to the side. This is often difficult. Ask the child to press his front knee outwards against your hand and also maintain balance. Augment his balance by offering manual resistance to his hips at the side, shoulder girdle at the side and shoulder and hip girdles at the same time.

Whilst on hands in half-kneeling and also in upright half-kneeling, grasp a support. Manual resistance may also be used. In addition head lift against resistance applied between his ears across the lower occiput helps to augment the stabilization.

Rising from prone to standing Once the half-kneeling position is assumed it should continue as a transitional position on the way to standing up. Assumption of half-kneeling takes place using the exercise in Figs 7.38–7.40. In Fig. 7.42 the therapist is helping the child place his foot flat on the ground. Figure 7.43 shows how to hold the knee and foot steady as the child rises. Another method is to hold the child's body under his chest whilst he controls his limbs, or for the child to grasp supports from the hands and knees position and pull himself up to standing via the half-kneeling position. You may also ask the child to rise against your hand pressing his lower back and pelvis as in Fig. 7.43.

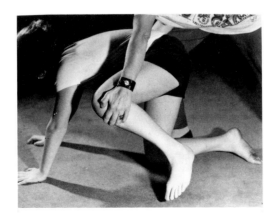

Fig. 7.42 Assumption of half-kneeling against the manual resistance or guidance of a therapist.

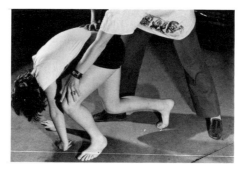

Fig. 7.43 Assumption of standing against manual resistance or guidance of a therapist.

Note The application of manual resistance must be done by physiotherapists as careful control of any abnormal overflow, the correct amount of resistance and technique of application is important.

See also other patterns of rising from prone in Fig. 7.184.

Weight taken on hands and feet and bear walk The child may place his hands on a low stool if he cannot easily reach the ground. Stabilization together with gentle passive stretching of tight hamstrings is carried out in this position. In addition the counterpoising exercises in Figs 7.38–7.40 should be done in this position and are illustrated in the development of standing at the 9–12 month developmental level (Figs 7.168, 7.169).

Stepping on hands and feet can be carried out using a stool on wheels, a low chair on sliding skis, with a sledge or stable wooden toy on wheels. Hold the child's thighs and knees straight and turned outward if there is any abnormal flexion-adduction-internal rotation. Give manual resistance to the stepping leg whilst holding the standing knee straight, to stretch tight hamstrings or increase the action of the fixators of the hip. Wearing knee gaiters for the bear walk or for slow upright stepping prevents the use of knee flexion *and* also activates the stabilizers (postural fixators) of the pelvic girdle. Joint compression through hips or knees of the standing leg also helps this stability.

Many normal children do not bear walk but the cerebral palsied and motor delayed child needs this motor activity for stabilization of shoulder girdle (lean on hands) and pelvic girdle, stretching of tight hamstrings, stretching of tight heel cords (heels kept flat on the ground) as well as the counterpoising of each limb as a step is taken.

Hyperextended knees may be treated in the bear walk (see Fig. 7.174).

Increasing stability of the hips is associated with a decrease of hyperextension of the knees which may be a compensation for lack of fixation at the hips.

Tilt reactions and saving reactions in limbs on hands and knees may be stimulated on a rocker board, inflatable mattress or thick soft sponge rubber (Fig. 7.44).

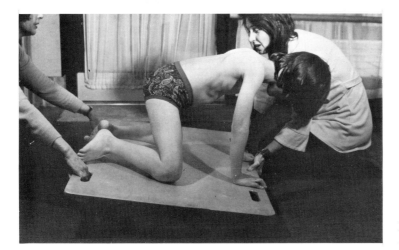

Fig. 7.44 Tilt responses activated on a rocker board.

Changes of posture from prone kneeling (on hands and knees) to sitting and back again, to prone lying and back again, to half-kneeling and back again and many other changes as in the righting reactions, should be trained at this level of development. See the development of sitting at this level. These activities overlap into all the other channels.

Problem of bunny hopping Reciprocal crawling rather than the continual bunny hopping of both knees forward should be present by this level. Unstable pelvis, excessive spasticity in hip and knee flexors and also habit prolong bunny hopping and aggravate these problems, as well as adding deformities of the feet. Discourage bunny hopping by offering other means of locomotion such as the prone board on casters for prone lying with hips and knees straight, a tricycle, pedal car, crawler and preferably walkers, with knees in gaiters, if necessary. Training children to bottom shuffle is also a good alternative and easily accepted by many children. The child sits with feet in front on the ground. He leans on his hands at his sides, presses his feet flat on the ground and stretches out his knees and moves along the ground, backwards, or forwards.

Encourage crawling on all surfaces, sand, grass, carpets, tiles, as well as using crawling on to a large step made with mattresses, wood or concrete, and climb in and out of boxes, cubby holes, through tunnels and under tables, etc.

Discourage crawling in children with tight hip and knee flexors and equinus feet. Practise pivot prone with feet in orthoses or use knee gaiters on prone trolleys.

Training upright kneeling This is discussed here as the child rises from prone positions to this position. Kneeling upright holding on to a support is expected at about 9–12 months whilst kneeling alone only at about 15 months in normal child development (Gesell 1971).

Do not use this position in children who persist with hip flexion, lordosis or hip-knee-dorsiflexion in this position. Control this by pressure against the extended hip and keeping the knees at right angles. The back is held straight by the child leaning his trunk against a sofa or holding the arms forward in flexion, elbows straight and lean or grasp a support. However all this may not really control every child's deformities.

Use upright kneeling if the abnormalities can be controlled (usually in athetoids and ataxics and motor delayed children) to develop vertical pelvic fixation and postural fixation of trunk on pelvis before standing supported is possible. Usually standing supported *is* possible if well controlled and is preferable. However, in children with deformities of the feet, plantigrade feet are not available for the standing position. Upright kneeling achievement in such a child confirms the need for surgery or plasters for the feet which are then preventing standing. Naturally knee flexors must also be checked for deformity.

Upright kneeling balance in kneel standing, knee walking sideways and forwards and backwards and kneeling on a rocker board may be useful in some children if for any reason these activities cannot be carried out in standing.

SUPINE DEVELOPMENT

The following main features should be developed:

Postural fixation of the shoulder girdle as the child holds the arm up in the air for reach, reach and grasp and other hand function and hand–eye coordination, beginning about 4 months normally when the hands are held in midline in, say, *hand regard*, at 5 months during reach for an object. (See the section on Basic arm and hand patterns for all levels of development under Development of hand function and also Table 7.6.)

Postural fixation of the pelvis as the child holds a leg up in the air, say, at 7 months in order to grasp his foot with his hand; at 5 months when a child *bridges* his hips off the surface *without* using back extensor spasm to do so.

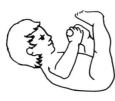

Fig. 7.45 Postural fixation and counterpoising of the limbs.

Counterpoising the limbs in the air (Fig. 7.45)   Children who cannot do this tip over when they are on their backs in water. Thus, holding a limb up in the air with absence of a hard surface increases a demand on the musculature needed for counterpoising, and reveals its inadequacy. Developmental level may be about 5–7 months when normal children hold their limbs steady in the air.

Rising reactions (Fig. 7.46)   These are probably the most important reactions or activities to be trained in supine development. Many abnormal postures and abnormal reactions are particularly obvious in supine. Training the child to get out of supine involves counteracting most of these reactions. This training seems to be preferable to spending time training the child's position in supine, except for severely immobile children who cannot manage this. Supine, *head rising* (righting) and the *overcoming of head lag* prepares and trains rising out of supine. Various *rolling-and-rising* reactions, e.g. roll and rise on to hands and knees, roll to prone and rise; roll half-way to side-lying or side-sitting; roll half-way and grasp a support and pull to sitting or standing, should be trained. If these are impossible, other patterns must be found as, say, in the athetoid child in Fig. 7.73. Rising is important as supine is a position of particular helplessness. Rising also contributes to a child's learning to get out of bed and turn at night.

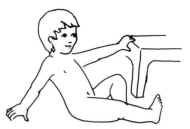

Fig. 7.46   Rising from supine.

Postural stabilization of the head (Fig. 7.47) is not head raising and requires special training. Head control is raising *and* holding of the head as well as head turning. Head holding is expected at 4–6 months normally, either in supine on the surface with head held off the surface, or, if the baby is held suspended horizontally in supine and he holds his head alone in this position, in midline.

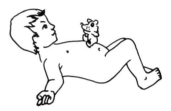

Fig. 7.47   Postural fixation of the head.

Note   Normal asymmetries, abnormal asymmetries and other aspects are discussed below. Pivoting on the back by movements of the arms and legs so that the child can move in circles may also be required in some children. *Tilt reactions* and *saving reactions* (Fig. 7.48) are less important in supine than in sitting and standing.

Treatment suggestions and daily care for all levels of development

SUPINE RISE TO SITTING AND DEVELOPMENT OF HEAD RIGHTING (RISING)

From 0–6 months normal development level   Help the child *to overcome head lag* using all or some of the following suggestions:

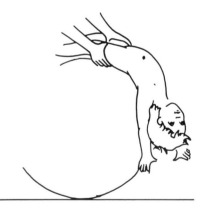

Fig. 7.48   Arms saving (parachute) reaction from supine.

(1)   First have the child lying half-way down against a back support or cushions, and encourage him to come up to sitting. Gradually decrease the back support so that eventually he raises his head and trunk from supine to sitting.
(2)   At first you will also have to hold his shoulders well forward, then later his upper arms and, as soon as possible, have him grasp your hands with his elbows straight. In these ways pull the child up to sitting, *waiting* for his own active head raise and later head and trunk (righting) raising. Some children bring their heads up first, their trunks follow. In others trunks may come up first and stimulate the head next (head-on-body righting; body-on-head righting).

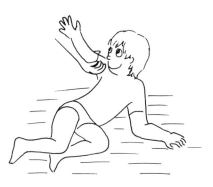

Fig. 7.61 Rising to sitting from side-lying.

supine position, have very poor head raising from supine, or require additional activity of the shoulder girdle muscles, back extensors, or arm elevation pattern (Fig. 7.61). Child in side-lying, hips and knees semiflexed, head forward and arm underneath the head with bent elbow. Lift the child's upper arm behind his occiput, turn the arm outward from the shoulder and gently pull this arm and thus the child up toward side-sitting, lean on elbow. Wait for his own active participation as he responds to gently pulling him up towards sitting. Later let him rise to side-sitting, lean on his hand instead of on his elbow. Check that his palm is down on the ground, his head is lifted up and sideways and his back is rotated and extended.

From 6–10 months normal developmental level Help the child *to rise* to sitting on his own in the following ways:

(1) Encourage his own head raise in supine by suspending him over the edge of a roll, your lap, a bed or a large ball. At first hold the child behind his shoulders, also place bells or toys on his tummy or feet so that the child is motivated to look up at them or at his toes (painted red if necessary!). Later, let him hang down over the edge of your lap, or the roll, and rock him upside down and call to him to raise his head.

(2) Supine to sitting should be carried out by helping the child to grasp a rope, parallel bars or vertical bars with one hand across his body, and pull himself to sitting in a diagonal direction with half-rotation of his trunk.

(3) Supine to sitting can be accomplished by the child if he holds a short pole or stick, held by you as well, with help to sitting. Help him avoid hunching his shoulders and excessively bending elbows and wrists to do this.

Remember the normal child will first come up to sitting from supine in a diagonal direction with a half-roll to one side and lean on one elbow or hand. He will only come straight up to sitting from supine much later, as this is an adult pattern seen in normal children over 4 years. Normally the child at the developmental level of 6–10 months may also roll over and rise to sitting. Rolling should also be trained for this.

PHYSIOTHERAPY SUGGESTIONS FOR ROLLING AND ROLL-AND-RISE

Rolling techniques will help the child to roll to side-lying where his hands might meet and he can see them. Correct rolling methods correct the abnormal positions of the legs and arms and can also stimulate head righting, decrease infantile neck righting and stimulate various body derotative and rotative patterns, and so learn to roll over to rise. He is then, in effect, using his body to turn in order to rise from supine. Some children need rolling for locomotion and exploring space. Some of the many methods available are:

Reflex rolling or primitive reactions   Turn the baby or child's head to one side and hold his jaw firmly. Press down and across the fifth intercostal space towards the *opposite* side. A reflex rotation will begin at the pelvis causing both knees and then one knee to flex up and over to the side of the child's occiput. This technique initiates rolling and prepares for roll-and-rise, also actively corrects leg adduction-extension, arm flexion, hand fisting and abnormal *roll-en-masse* (Fig. 7.62), and *frog position*.

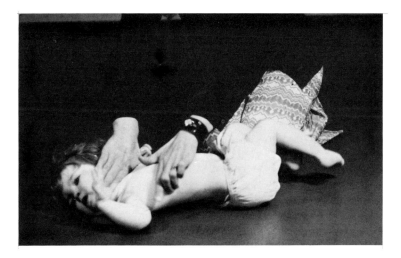

Fig. 7.62   Reflex rolling.

Side-lying   Rotate the child's shoulder girdle forward while rotating his pelvis back. Change to rotation of the shoulder backward and pelvis forward, and vice versa (Figs 7.63, 7.64). If speed is correct and the rotary stretch on the trunk adequate, these *counter rotations* stimulate an active response in the child's shoulder or pelvis or in both areas. This also treats the rolling *in one piece* as seen, say, in the neck righting reaction. If rotation of the shoulder girdle is possible against some manual resistance, there is often an associated head raising with the rotation. Rotation of the girdles, pelvic/shoulder, not only facilitates rolling but also initiates arm movements and leg movements. Train shoulder rotation backwards as a preliminary to pulling the arm out from underneath the body in those children who get their arm caught in rolling over.

Supine. Leg patterns
(1)   Bend both the child's knees across to the opposite side whilst rotating and holding his upper shoulder back. Release his shoulders and an active roll of the upper trunk follows. This roll might be manually resisted at the shoulder as well, but check that correct

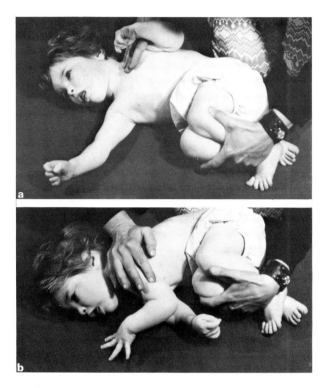

Fig. 7.63 Using knees to rotate pelvis in side-lying.

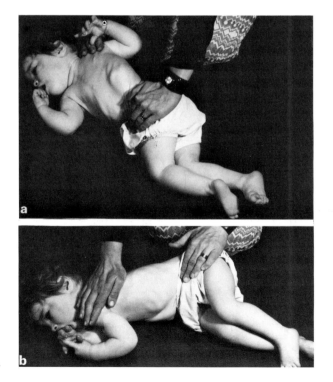

Fig. 7.64 Rotation of the shoulder girdles and pelvic girdles.

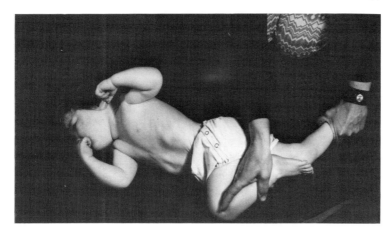

Fig. 7.65 Supine, leg patterns.

resistance is given so that a full flexion spasm does *not* occur (Fig. 7.63).

(2) Stretch one of the child's legs into extension-abduction and then stimulate this leg to move to flexion-adduction to the opposite side. Wait for his upper trunk to roll over bringing the arm across (Fig. 7.65). A retraction of the shoulder often delays or even prevents the arm coming over within the child's roll from supine to prone. If possible facilitate leg flexion-adduction against resistance given at the knee and thigh. This shows him an active leg pattern.

Arm patterns

(1) Bring the child's arm from his side in shoulder extension-abduction-internal rotation and across his body to flexion-adduction-external rotation (child's palm must be towards his face) (Fig. 7.66). Wait for him to turn his head, trunk and legs. The therapist may carry this out passively, use stretch and resistance or motivate a baby to reach for a toy on the opposite side of the moving arm.

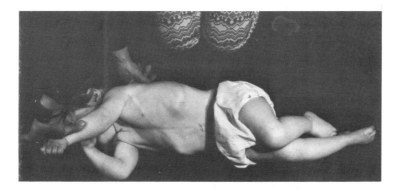

Fig. 7.66 Supine, arm patterns.

(2)   Elevate and hold both the child's arms above his head in supine or in prone. Bring one arm across to the other to stimulate the child's automatic roll.

(3)   If the underneath arm gets caught, hold it straight above his head.

Note

(1)   Prone-supine rolling: use the arm or leg pattern of extension-rotation.

(2)   During rolling over, various leg patterns are themselves stimulated, i.e. leg flexes over with the roll from supine to prone in some children. In others the child may use the leg to *push-off* in an extended-abducted pattern (Fig. 7.67). During the roll from prone to supine, some children extend and abduct the upper leg. Other children flex the upper leg as they roll. Similarly arm patterns vary. The therapist must select the technique according to the reaction she wishes to obtain.

(3)   Combinations of head, arm and leg patterns also vary.

(4)   All rolling patterns relax a stiff child.

Head patterns   Raise the child's head into flexion-rotation and wait for him to follow with rolling towards the side to which his face is rotated. Hold his head lightly as he rolls. You may have to hold his chin up as he reaches prone. Resisted head flexion-rotation may be used as well in

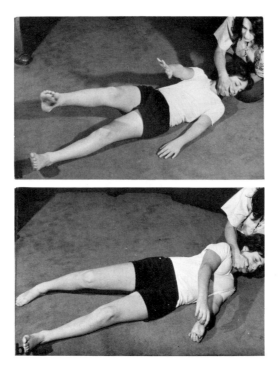

Fig. 7.67   Head pattern to stimulate rolling. *Note* limb reaction a, b.

children who have good head control and respond with rolling in their waist and not en-masse. Prone to supine rolling is carried out with head raise to extension-rotation. The arm patterns above may also provoke the head patterns. Some children may use an arm to push-off together with head patterns (Fig. 7.67).

Rolling to instructions   *Head, arm or leg* patterns may be carried over from the facilitation techniques by some intelligent children. Instructions used for say: *prone lying* with arms overhead 'lift your head and one (right) arm up and back as far as possible', 'roll over'; 'lift your leg up and back, over to the other side', 'roll over'.

Supine lying   'Bend one knee right across to the other side as far as it will go', 'roll over'; 'grasp your hands and stretch your elbows – bring both arms over to one side as far as possible', 'roll over'; 'lift your head and look over to one side as far as possible', 'roll over'.

TREATMENT SUGGESTIONS AND DAILY CARE FOR ROLLING AND RISING

Rolling
(1)   Place the child on his back, on his side or on his stomach (with face and neck over the edge) on a blanket. Hold each end of the blanket – two adults may be needed – and suspend the child in the blanket just off the ground. Tip the child gently from side to side, waiting for him to complete his roll over. If he cannot do this himself you can roll him in the blanket until he picks up the rolling motion himself. *Do not* do this with a child who arches his back or overextends when in prone position. Keep repeating this roll sideways in suspension in supine with his head, shoulders and hips bent. Also suspend the child in a hammock, if arching persists in supine position.
(2)   Child lying on his back – bend one hip and knee well over to the opposite side and wait for him to complete the roll over (Fig. 7.65).
(3)   Bring one of his arms over to the opposite side with the palm of his hand towards his face, or offer him a toy he likes on the opposite side, this may lead to a roll over (Fig. 7.66). Offer him a toy for rolling from side-lying or from prone.
(4)   Child lying on his stomach – bring his hip and pelvis, or his shoulders, back and towards the opposite side and encourage rolling. Some children may push off on one hand to help roll from prone to supine, or rise on to their lower arms underneath their bodies.
(5)   Child in prone or supine on a soft thick sponge rubber mattress or inflatable bed. Press down on one side of his body so that he tips over towards you and rolls. Rolling on such surfaces is often easier as he does not get *stuck* with his arm caught under his body. At first it is necessary to place the arm, which gets caught underneath, above his head.

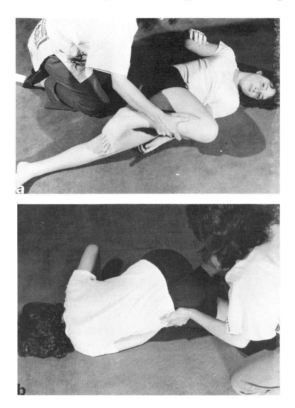

Fig. 7.68   Roll-to-rise onto hands and knees. *Note* many methods exist for this but must be demonstrated clinically.

(6)   Encourage rolling on all surfaces, floors, carpets, grass and sand. Make an incline with a pile of mattresses or sponge rubber, or place the child on the top of a slight mound of grass or sand and let gravity help him roll downhill on his own.

(7)   If a child can roll over *wait* for him to do so. In addition train him to roll over from his back to his stomach and then to get up on to his hands and knees (as described in prone development, 3–6 months level or Fig. 7.68a,b).

Stages in supine development

0–3 Months normal developmental level

COMMON PROBLEMS

Delay in gradual overcoming of head lag on pull to sitting. Inability to lift hand to mouth.

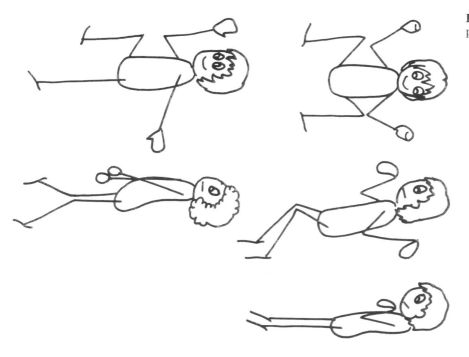

Fig. 7.69 Some abnormal patterns in supine.

Abormal performance (Fig. 7.69) Opisthotonus, or excessive extension of either head, shoulder girdle, back and legs or all of them. Some arch into opisthotonus in infancy but become floppy later. Floppy babies may have intermittent extensor spasms of head, spine and hips. They may also lie in frog positions with the legs flexed-abducted-externally rotated, arms limp at their sides or in shoulder abduction, elbow flexion, hands open or closed. Apparently normal flexion positions may also be present in babies who later become spastic. Kicking of legs begins but may be simultaneous with abnormal asymmetry in that one leg flexes, abducts and sometimes externally rotates, while the other flexes, adducts and sometimes internally rotates, or one may kick more vigorously than the other. This asymmetry may become so great that the legs look *windswept* to one side, especially when kicking stops. Hip dislocation is threatening in the adducted-internally rotated leg. Persistent head turning to one side may occur. Pelvic obliquity and scoliosis may appear.

Reflex reactions Normally these include grasp reflex, Moro reaction, asymmetrical tonic neck reaction, leg crossed extensor reflex, withdrawal reflex, neck righting reaction. On passively pulling the child to sitting, his legs should flex-adduct and, by the next 3–6 months level, flex-abduct. A response of extension-adduction of the legs is abnormal. Some cerebral palsied children even extend the hips so much that their hips come well off the surface. Others cannot *fix* their bottom on a surface and slide easily on it.

See section on Physiotherapy suggestions for rolling and roll-and-rise as a child can only respond on an automatic level at this stage. Continue into next stage of development, then add more advanced methods.

TREATMENT SUGGESTIONS AND DAILY CARE

(1)   See Supine rise to sitting and development of head righting (rising), from 0–6 months.
(2)   Bring a child's arms well forward and turn them out from his shoulders, so that both hands touch your face, or make him touch his own hands, mouth, chest or abdomen naming these body parts. Stimulate visually and with noises in the centre to encourage his head holding in the centre and hands should make contact with bells or musical toys dangling in the midline.
(3)   Eye-to-eye contact with your eyes parallel to his, at first in the centre. Then stimulate him to follow sounds, lights and mobiles from side-to-side (see development of hand function in Table 7.6).
(4)   *Abnormal reflex reactions and abnormal performance* are modified as follows:
   • *Discourage* supine if the child has asymmetrical tonic neck reaction after 4 months, excessive Moro after 6 months or has extensor spasms. It is better that the child is in prone or sitting positions selected according to his level of development. Head should be in the centre and both arms held parallel and forward at the shoulder level in these positions. If supine is inevitable during periods in the day, hold the child's head up into flexion in the hollow of a large cushion; use a hammock (Fig. 7.70). This overcomes the head falling or pressing back into extension. Head flexion often diminishes the ATNR, Moro or extensor thrusts. In this position hold his arms symmetrical (parallel) and brought well (flexed) forward at the shoulders. Motivate these symmetrical arm movements with toys, mobiles and so on.
   • Excessively extended children should be flexed at head, shoulders and hips in side-lying or supine (Fig. 7.70). The severely extended child, especially if the arms are always at the sides with retracted shoulders and bent elbows, should be kept in side-lying with support from pillows or a *side-lying board* (Fig. 7.70c) so that his hands will be able to meet and so that he can see them, so that they can touch his mouth and later reach for toys in front of him (5 months' level). Place a toy between his hands that can easily be grasped (see Hand function), later train

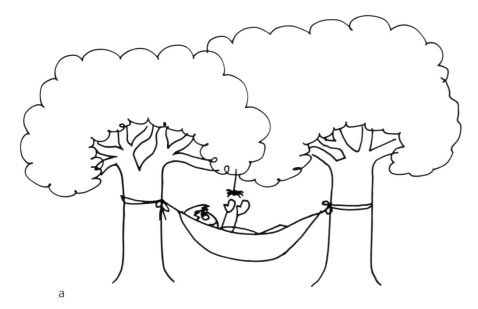

a

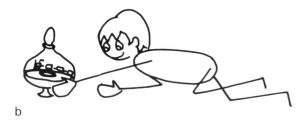

b

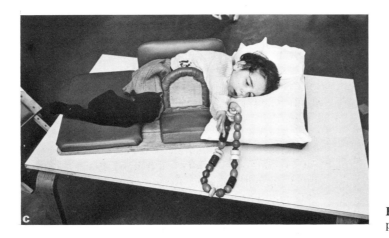

Fig. 7.70   Some corrective positions.

him to lie on his side alone. Show the child how to balance in side-lying with one leg on top of the other, as well as one in front of the other.

- For a child with abnormally straight legs, pressed together and turned in, use abduction pants. For frog position use sandbags to keep the legs together as you train rising or sitting or talk to the child in supine. Pants that are well stitched down the centre can be used to bring the legs together in lying. Sometimes arms held down and in front stimulate legs coming together.
- Persistent head turning should be discouraged by getting the child to look the other way. His bed should be on the opposite side of the room, offer toys, communication and even food from the side towards which the child rarely turns. Carry the child so that he can also look to the side which is not usually preferred. The physiotherapist must check that the child does not have a torticollis which requires stretching or even an operation. Plagiocephaly may accompany head turning. This strong head turning or preference has been observed in some babies who were really normal (Robson 1970).
- See therapy for grasp reflex in stages of hand function development, 0–3 months' and 3–5 months' levels, Moro in the Development of sitting, crossed extensor pattern, withdrawal pattern, in Development of standing, neck righting pattern in Rolling Techniques (Leg patterns, Arm patterns and Side-lying).
- Abnormal synergies, i.e. leg extension-adduction-internal rotation are best corrected in the creeping patterns at this level in prone development. If prone development is not indicated in the particular child, train reciprocal leg movement in supine. Carry out active assisted full range of reciprocal motion. Hold the child's knees and bend one hip and knee up and out, holding the other leg straight and turned out. Change the motion by bringing the bent leg down as you move the straight leg up into flexion (Fig. 7.71).

4–6 Months normal development level

COMMON PROBLEMS

Delay in acquisition of symmetry, in keeping head in the centre, in bringing the arms together and in hand regard. Delay in the disappearance of head lag and in acquiring ability to raise the head off the bed. The child is unable to *bridge* his hips off the floor, unable to reach for a toy (see Hand function, Table 7.6).

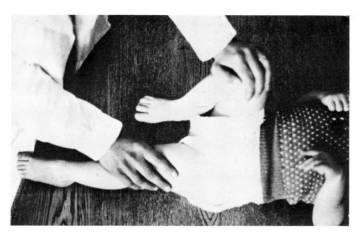

Fig. 7.71 Assisted active reciprocal motion. Hold one leg well down while fully flexing the other. Point knees outward. Use song for slow rhythm.

Abnormal performance Flexed legs now abnormally extend-adduct and internally rotate in many spastic children in lying supine and when brought from supine to sitting position. Normally legs flex-abduct and externally rotate at this level. Presence of clenched hands (see arm function). Abnormal absence of isolated foot movements or knee movements, as these only occur as part of 'mass patterns'. Abnormal anterior pelvic tilt.

Reflex reactions May not be developing body derotation. Reflexes of 0–6 months level may not be disappearing.

TREATMENT SUGGESTIONS AND DAILY CARE

(1) See Hand function (Table 7.6).
(2) See rise up to sitting and rolling techniques, especially rolling with rotation or turning at the child's waist line during a roll over.

PHYSIOTHERAPY SUGGESTIONS

Arm reach Child in side-lying and progress to supine. Facilitate arm patterns of flexion-adduction-external rotation with straight elbow and also with bent elbow, so that hands touch the child's mouth. Carry this out as a unilateral pattern in side-lying and as a bilateral pattern in supine (see Hand function, Fig. 7.199). Place attractive objects in positions, near a child, which activate these arm patterns. His lack of shoulder girdle stability may cause compensatory shoulder hunching and manual guidance is given to help him control this.

Bridging (Fig. 7.72) Hold the child's feet flat on the floor. He raises his hips to let a toy go *under the bridge*. Check that this is *not done* by using

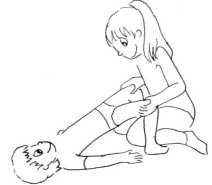

Fig. 7.72 Bridging.

a lumbar lordosis. Check that arms do not flex up into abnormal postures. Hold the 'bridge' steady while the wind tries to 'blow it over'. On this instruction the therapist gives manual resistance at the side of the child's pelvis, or on the anterior superior iliac spines, or one hand in front and one behind to rotate his pelvis. The child must maintain the stability of the bridge as far as possible. A pillow under his hips may help initially as he learns to maintain control against your manual pressure and resistance.

Note Semi-bridging and moving backwards is a form of locomotion used by some athetoid and more rarely by spastic children. However, this is often abnormal as it includes excessive hypertonic arching in the head and back and retraction of the shoulder. This should be discouraged and another form of locomotion offered to the child.

6–9 Months normal motor developmental level

COMMON PROBLEMS

Delay in grasping feet with legs in the air. The child is unable to roll over or pull himself towards sitting.

Abnormal performance He cannot lie straight with arms and legs extended or with legs abducted-extended-externally rotated. A variety of abnormal postures may be seen including asymmetry of head, trunk or limbs or all of these. Normally, the pull-to-sit should provoke extension-abduction of legs. Anterior pelvic tilt may persist abnormally.

Abnormal rolling patterns may be roll, leading with head and arms but with legs stiff and straight or passive; roll, using legs but upper arm bent and retracted at the shoulder; roll, using a *flexion into a ball*, or using an arching of the back and head to roll over. No rotation at the child's waist (body rotative pattern), i.e. either rolling in one piece or using the abnormal total flexion or extension; roll to one side only, in say hemiplegia, towards the affected side only, using the unaffected side to carry out the roll over, or in say quadriplegia using the less affected side to carry out the roll, or in others, simply being unable to roll to a particular side.

TREATMENT SUGGESTIONS AND DAILY CARE

(1) See, rising to sitting, 6–10 months level, Rolling Techniques (see sections on Rolling to instructions and Treatment suggestions and daily care for rolling and rising). Use arm and leg patterns against manual resistance at this stage. See also Table 7.6 for a child's development of hand function. At this stage a child may show his own strategies of rising (see Figs 7.73 and 7.74). See also the section in Chapter 4 on A child's own goals and strategies.

(2) Have the child in supine and help him to hold one or both of his feet. Turn his hips and knees outward and bend his leg so his foot is touching his hand. Gently stretch his knee and lift his leg so that he can reach for, look at and also grasp his feet and hold them. First

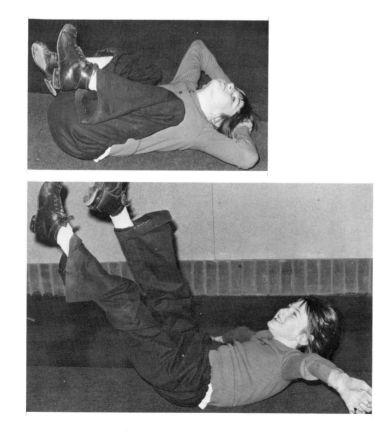

Fig. 7.73 Athetoid girl using her own method of rising (bend knees to chest and swing up to sitting, or grasp clothes and pull up to sitting).

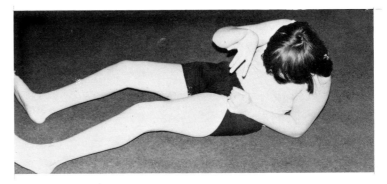

Fig. 7.74 Spastic boy using his own method of rising to sitting. He grasps his clothes and pulls himself up alone.

bend his hips and lift his bottom off the bed if he is unable to reach. The child must also actively bend his hip and knee to his chest so that the full hip flexion is attained. Ask him to 'kiss his knee', 'to pull his sock or shoe off his toes' or to 'hug his knees to his chest'. Play 'peek-a-boo' as he opens and closes his ankles and feet above his face. All these actions help overcome abnormal pelvic anterior tilt and activate abdominals.

Note that no further developmental training is needed in supine as, from 10 months onward the child normally *dislikes* lying supine and persists in rolling out of this position or pulling up to sitting.

(3) Having trained the child to rise from supine to sitting *does not mean he can sit*. See Development of Sitting (Figs 7.80–7.93) which should be trained at the same time as Supine Development. Levels of development of sitting and rise to sitting may be at different motor ages.

(4) Practise rising to sitting and rolling in order to get out of bed.

DEVELOPMENT OF SITTING

The following main aspects should be developed:

Postural fixation of the head or vertical head control. Normally developed by 3 months.

Head righting or rising to the vertical position. Normally developed by 3 months.

Postural fixation of the head and the trunk (Fig. 7.75). Normally developed by 3–6 months and independent by 9 months.

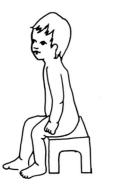

Fig. 7.75 Postural fixation.

Head and trunk righting or rising from sitting, leaning or slumped forward, backward or sideways, to upright sitting (Fig. 7.76) Normally developed between 3–12 months depending upon the positions and support given to the child.

Note Rising to sitting from supine, see Supine development, and from prone, see Prone development. Rising from sitting to standing, see Development of standing and walking.

Postural fixation of the shoulder girdle Normally developed by 3–6 months. This is associated with a reinforcement of fixation of the head and also with the use of the arms for supports in sitting. Use of hands also activates shoulder girdle stabilization.

Postural fixation of head on trunk and trunk on pelvis. Normally developed by 6 months with support and independently with head and trunk by 9 months.

Sitting counterpoising head, arm, trunk and leg movements (Fig. 7.77). Normally developed by 6–12 months (see also Development of hand function and Dressing and feeding). Postural control cannot be separated from hand function.

Tilt reactions (Fig. 7.78) When the child is tilted sideways, forwards or backwards (his bottom is tilted off the horizontal). Normally developed by 9–12 months.

Saving reactions (Fig. 7.79) and propping reactions if the child falls. Normally developed forward by about 5–7 months, sideways by about 9 months and backward by about 12 months.

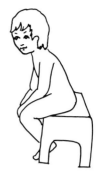

Fig. 7.76 Rising to upright sitting and reverse.

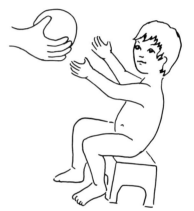

Fig. 7.77 Counterpoising.

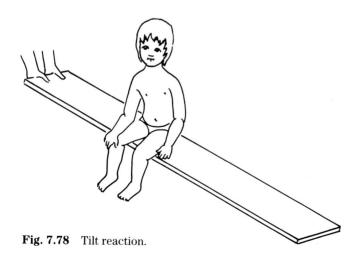

Fig. 7.78 Tilt reaction.

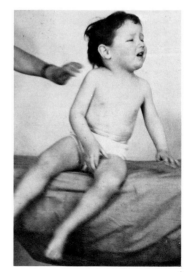

Fig. 7.79 Saving reactions in the arms and legs.

Stages in development of sitting (Fig. 7.80–7.93)

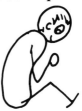

Fig. 7.80 Sitting head uncontrolled, flexion in total child (*0–3 months*).

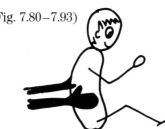

Fig. 7.81 Decrease of flexion, vertical head control develops (*0–3 months*).

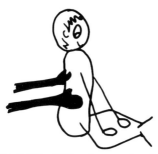

Fig. 7.82 Sitting lean on hands, flattening of upper back develops, lumbar kyphosis still present (*4–6 months*).

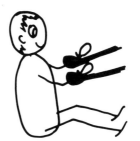

Fig. 7.83 Sitting with less support, back straighter, legs straighter, turning out and apart (*4–6 months*).

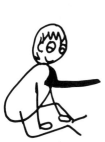

Fig. 7.84 Sitting lean on hands, hips flexed-abducted-externally rotated. Less support and without support (*4–6 months*).

Fig. 7.85 Sitting in baby chair with back and sides supporting or propped on a pillow support (*4–6 months*).

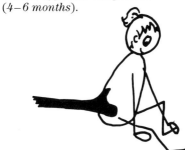

Fig. 7.86 Sitting lean on hands and lift one hand to play, with feet or a toy (*6–9 months*).

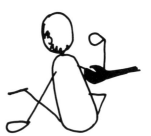

Fig. 7.87 Saving reactions and propping in arms (*6–9 months*). Tilt reactions begin.

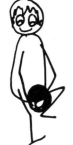

Fig. 7.88 Sitting alone on the ground (*6–9 months*).

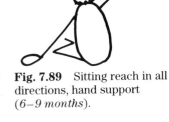

Fig. 7.89 Sitting reach in all directions, hand support (*6–9 months*).

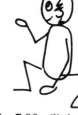

Fig. 7.90 Sitting turn to play reach, no hand support (*9–12 months*).

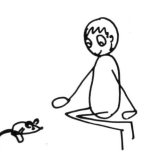

Fig. 7.91 Sitting in various positions (*9–12 months*). Pivot in sitting.

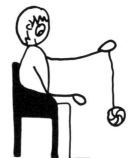

Fig. 7.92 Sitting in a chair and play, sit alone in regular chair on a stool (*9–12 months*).

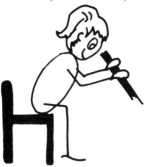

Fig. 7.93 Rising out of sitting and getting into all sitting positions. Tilt reactions complete (*9–12 months*).

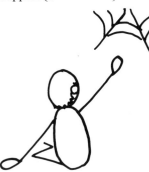

Abnormal postures in sitting at all levels of development (Fig. 7.94)

These may be due to:

(1) Absence of the above postural mechanisms and compensatory abnormal postures to obtain balance.
(2) Presence of hypertonus.
(3) Attempts by an older child to control disrupting involuntary movements.
(4) Use of incorrect size and type of chairs, tables, pushchairs, wheelchairs and continual placement of child in only one or more poor sitting positions.
(5) Prolonged sitting in one special chair beyond two hours, even if positions are corrected.

Absence of postural stabilization results in a child falling backwards or leaning back as he slides out of the seat of his chair. The normal postural stabilization holds the hips at right angles to the trunk as the pelvis and trunk are stabilized. In development the back is first rounded with pelvis

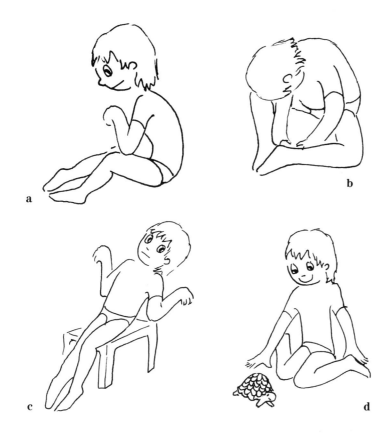

Fig. 7.94 a,b,c and d Some abnormal postures in sitting.

tilted backwards and subsequently the back straightens with pelvis tilting towards the front. Delay in postural stabilization is compensated for by various abnormal postures. These may lead to deformities. Abnormal postures may be:

(1) Head and trunk flex on semi-extended hips in *sacral sitting* (Fig. 7.94a and b). Arms may flex and shoulders hunch tensely as a child avoids falling by grasping a support near his body. He may instead prop on his fists for support with his arms tensely internally rotated with straight elbows. He may maintain his flexed position without hand support but has to hyperextend his neck to avoid falling forward and in order to look up.

(2) When a child leans back against a chair, his arms may be held up in abduction at his sides with shoulders hunched, protracted or retracted (Fig. 7.94c). He may instead elevate his arms forwards at 45–90° in the air with elbows straight, shoulders hunched in an effort to counterbalance his backward fall or extensor thrust. His feet may plantar flex to reach the ground for support or if the ground is near enough his toes flex to 'hold on' and his feet may press into valgus for support (Fig. 7.94c).

(3) A child sitting on a bed, the floor or on a chair which is too high may adduct and internally rotate his semi-extended hips with straight or bent knees. He may strongly bend his knees over the edge of the chair, twisting his legs around the front legs of the chair to avoid falling.

(4) Sitting on the floor with his bottom between his feet and his legs internally rotated and flexed is often seen in a child with cerebral palsy *W sitting* (Fig. 7.94d). This is one way in which an unstable child can stabilize his pelvis and develop head and trunk control and hand function. Although this posture is seen in able-bodied children, it is not held for the many long periods which children with cerebral palsy persist in doing. Deformities of hip, knee and feet may develop unless there is more variety in floor sitting. Tailor sitting and long sitting with legs straight in front of a child also reveal very rounded backs and difficulty in using hands and reaching.

(5) Some children stabilize better on one side of their hips or trunk and prefer to sit sideways on to one buttock. This is obvious in children with hemiplegia but also when there are *windswept* legs to one side (Fig. 7.95). Scolioses may result from persistent asymmetrical weight bearing in sitting. If a child can only use one hand or one visual field this also aggravates or causes postural stabilization and counter-poising on one side.

ABNORMAL SITTING POSTURES IN SPASTIC (HYPERTONIC) CHILDREN

If the child is also hypertonic, he will assume the same postures already

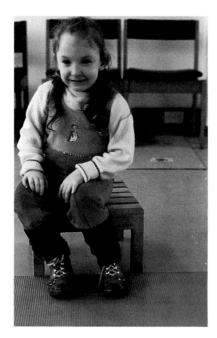

Fig. 7.95 Sitting with 'windswept' legs to one side. A mild example which may be much more severe in other children.

described, but the shortened or shortening spastic or rigid muscles maintain or augment these abnormal postures, as well as others. Thus prolonged sitting in any one position is particularly dangerous as it causes deformity and so disabling influences on the development of standing and walking and hand function development.

The above postures associated with the tightness of spastic muscles will be seen as:

(1) Stiff extension so that the child cannot be flexed into the sitting position unless special methods are used. Some children can overcome their *extensor thrusts* or extensor hypertonus by using flexor hypertonus and sitting in excessive flexion.

(2) Some severely extended children may collapse into a flexion spasm or flexion and floppiness once the extensor hypertonus or spasm is overcome by the therapist. No sitting is possible in either position, showing absence of postural mechanisms.

(3) Most children achieve a position somewhere between full flexion or extension. The falling backward and extensor thrust seem to remain *in the hips* but trunk flexes with arms and head extends, legs assume various postures depending on the distribution of the spasticity in each child. Trunk, head and arms also vary according to the child. Some children have hypertonus in the trunk, often on one side only. Scoliosis together with torticollis may be present.

(4) Tight hamstrings are often present in hypertonic children. The pelvis

is tilted back in sitting by the pull of the tight hamstrings. If the knees are extended as in long-sitting on the floor (Fig. 7.94a) the child may fall backward as his hamstrings do not allow this full extension. Many children can maintain long-sit with their pelvis tipped back in sacral sitting with a round back if they semiflex at the knees. On a chair, the child's knees can bend fully and this often tips the pelvis back into position for upright sitting with the child's weight on his tuberosities and not on his sacrum.

Knee flexion deformities are particularly threatening in these children, especially if they have prolonged sitting on chairs, where they find sitting so much easier.

Treatment and daily care at all levels of development

PRACTICAL SUGGESTIONS FOR ABNORMAL POSTURES AND BALANCE

Abnormal postures are corrected as actively as possible. Special corrections may be given with special chairs (adaptive seating) – see below.

Kyphosis Try active arm patterns involving elevation, as well as the general development of postural alignment and stabilization of head, trunk and pelvis in sitting and other channels of development (see the section on Basic arm and hand patterns for all levels of development under Development of hand function).

Scoliosis Make sure the child sits on both his buttocks. Reaching overhead is helpful on the side of the concavity. Sandbags or a roll of towels on his table under his forearm on the side of the concavity, or under the buttock on either the side of the concavity or convexity, should be tried to discover which props him into a more upright position.

Abnormal postures of arms, trunk, head, legs are often corrected at the same time if the child sits on *both* his ischial tuberosities, leans forward from his hips, back straight to lean on his open hands with elbows held straight. Legs should be held apart and turned outward if they adduct. When knees are always in flexion, then use knee gaiters and sitting raised just off the floor if his back rounds, in preference to chair sitting. Feet should be flat on the ground if the child sits on a chair. Foot supports are essential if he is on a high chair (see Fig. 7.96). Correction of equinus feet, as discussed in Chapter 9, is important as this provides plantigrade feet as extra supports for sitting balance.

Some ideas to correct leg postures include sitting with any adducted legs apart and turned out on either side of large toys, a box of toys, bowl of sand or water, a small drum, straddling rolls, soft toys, the corner of the

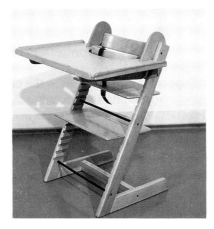

Fig. 7.96 Trip-trap chair.

bed or chair, and across your hip or thigh. Do not have the child straddle anything of too great a diameter as he then increases hip internal rotation with excessive abduction of his hips. Abduction splints may have to be worn during sitting for better hip posture (see Fig. 5 in Appendix). Tailor-sitting or side-sitting are preferable to sitting between his knees (Fig. 7.134), but should also be avoided if there is too much flexion in the child's hips and knees as well as abnormal adduction and internal rotation. Feet need to also be checked in case they deform in these sitting positions. Avoid side-sitting to a windswept postural preference, if present.

Avoid prolonged sitting especially if there is tightness of hip and knee flexors. Encourage standing up and standing positions or prone lying instead.

Excessive hip, trunk and head extension is corrected within the postures above, as well as having the child learn to sit on low chairs, kneel sit, sit in the corner of the sofa, or room, and into various special seating (see below). Carry the child in full flexion, to counteract severe extension and just before he is placed into his special *flexion chairs* – see below and Fig. 8.8.

Remember that when the child leans forward from his hips to reach his toys, feet or prop himself on his hands, he should lean from his hip joint. He avoids rounding his back instead of flexing in his hip. Help him by pressing your hand on the small of his back, if he cannot manage alone. Also make sure that the pull of tight hamstrings is not causing this and whether a small raise on to a platform for his floor seat is required. This is especially necessary if he is wearing knee extension splints. Sitting on a thick cushion, or sponge on the floor, may also improve posture of his back. If he sits on a forward-downward tilt on a wedge it may straighten his back.

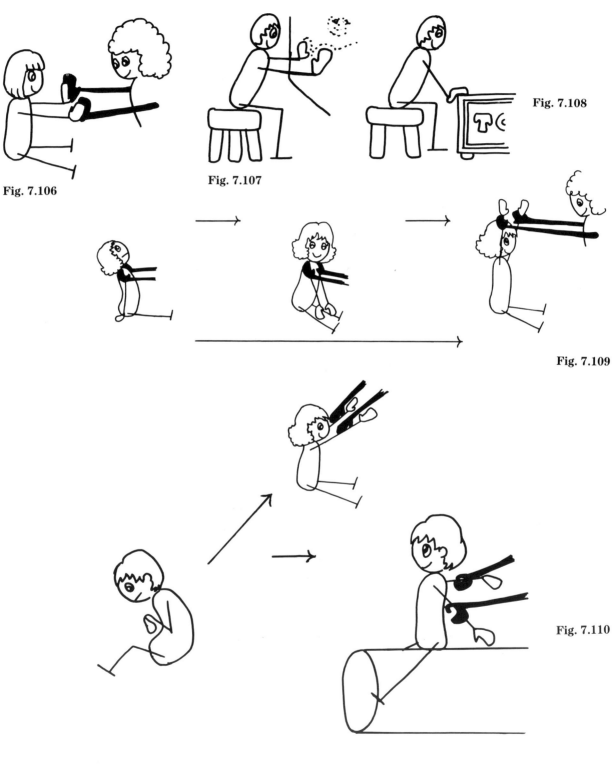

Fig. 7.106

Fig. 7.107

Fig. 7.108

Fig. 7.109

Fig. 7.110

Child takes weight on forearms (Fig. 7.102). If child presses his arms to his chest use a roll of towels or sponge wedge to avoid this. Joint compression through shoulders or head may also be used.

Child is helped to lean on his forearms into adult's hands (Fig. 7.103). Adult reinforces this joint compression by pushing child's upper arm into his shoulder joint. Head and trunk control are thus activated within social interaction.

Visual and auditory stimuli at child's eye level for vertical head and trunk control in sitting (Fig. 7.104). Upright posture is encouraged.

Sitting grasping a pole, edge of a table or adult's hands (Fig. 7.105). Elbows should be straight and symmetrical. The support may be grasped with his arms at shoulder level, below shoulder level or above shoulder level. Child leans against table edge at lower levels of development (0–6 months).

Child pushes his open hands against adult's hands with wrists dorsiflexed (Fig. 7.106).

Child may also push against wall, make *hand prints* on powdered or soaped mirror or push firm toy to make a sound (Fig. 7.107). Trunk support may be given by leaning against a table edge or manually at 0–6 months level.

Child leans on hands on floor, child on a chair can lean on his hands (Fig. 7.108).

Stimulate head righting by bringing his shoulders forward and then take his upper arms, turn them out and elevate them to hold a toy in front of him or for dressing (Fig. 7.109). Make sure he tips his head forward when clothes are put over his head.

In Fig. 7.110 stimulate head righting by pulling shoulder girdle backwards or arms back against your hands to lean back on his hands with a straight back.

Manual resistance may be given at the child's shoulder on its lateral aspect or anteroposterior aspect (Fig. 7.111). This reinforces head fixation, shoulder girdle fixation (stability). Do this also with the child leaning on forearms (Fig. 7.102), on hands (Fig. 7.101), or grasping a support.

Note: Give the correct amount of resistance so that abnormal reactions are not provoked in legs or body.

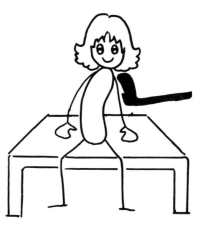

Fig. 7.111

CHAIRS AND TABLES

Special chairs (adaptive seating) are selected according to the child's developmental level to:

(1) Train sitting.
(2) Correct abnormal postures.
(3) Provide stimulation in the upright position to develop a child's social, visual and hearing abilities.

(4)   Develop hand function in the *upright* position of *supported* sitting. Meanwhile training of sitting balance must continue and be associated with hand function as soon as possible. (See Basic arm and hand patterns for all levels of development under Development of hand function.)

Regular chairs are used:

(1)   To increase development of sitting balance and independent good posture.
(2)   To develop hand function together with sitting balance.
(3)   To make standing up from sitting possible.

Measurements   If chairs are not of the correct measurements for the child they can obstruct the development of sitting, cause or increase abnormal postures and prevent hand function (Fig. 7.112). Only use an armrest if that support is needed. The back rest is 100° to seat. Table should be up to the height of child's waist or higher if he lacks trunk control. There should be a *large* area of work space.

If the chair is *too high* the child will find lack of foot support for his dangling feet disturbing to his poor sitting balance. Plantarflexed feet may become plantarflexion deformity. If the chair is *too wide* the child may take more weight on one side as he slumps to that side. The lateral lean or slumping decreases balance and may lead to scoliosis. Place rolls of towel, sponge-covered blocks, sandbags or magazines to decrease a chair which is too wide. The seat could be made to fit his buttocks. If the

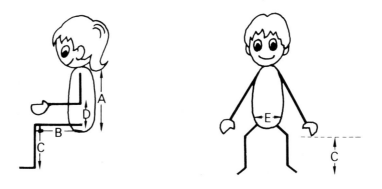

A	Height of backrest
B	Seat depth
C	Seat to floor
D	Armrest height
E	Seat width

Fig. 7.112

chair seat is *too short* the child may not be able to balance without support to his thighs. His feet may twist or curl around the chair legs in his efforts to balance. Deformity of his feet and of flexed, adducted internally rotated knees may be encouraged. If the chair seat is *too long* he may slump backwards to the back support and increase hip extension, adduction and internal rotation, knee extension and plantarflexion or hip extension adduction, semiflexion of the knees and plantarflexion of his feet. Rounding of the back is inevitable. In all the above situations the child's hand function is made impossible or difficult.

EVALUATING A CHAIR FOR A CHILD

Most therapists use trial and error to assess which chair and table is most suitable for an individual child. Research continues among therapists and bioengineers to clarify when particular designs are indicated for specific problems. Controversy still exists between different workers. The studies of the following are among many others which can guide clinical therapists: Trefler *et al.* 1978; Nwaobi *et al.* 1983, 1987; Mulcahy *et al.* 1988; Myhr & von der Wendt 1990; McCarthy 1992 (seating). Controversy about seating may arise when clinicians are really comparing children at different stages of development of quiet sitting versus sitting for hand function, vision and communication or for balance training. An *assessment chair* with different elements which can be removed according to each child helps to make decisions as to which chair is suitable. Try this with a child in quiet sitting and during functions and where relevant during transport. Bardsley, in a chapter in Eckersley (1993), describes an assessment chair which affects details of design which can be custom made if this is financially feasible. Zacharkow (1988) has written a book with useful suggestions for seating.

Potential seat elements (Fig. 7.113a–d)

There is an increasing range of seating systems for children produced by different manufacturers as well as custom made individual seating and the use of orthotics for desirable sitting positions. For most mild and moderately involved children with physical disabilities, for babies and for developmentally delayed children, mass produced regular chairs and tables are suitable. A few modifications with foot rests and foam pieces or firm cushions can be used to obtain the desirable posture in each child.

General considerations in selecting a chair
(1) Parents and child find the chair aesthetically acceptable.
(2) The chair should be comfortable not only during quiet sitting but also when a child moves his head, body and arms. It should be comfortable and safe when the chair is moved from place to place.

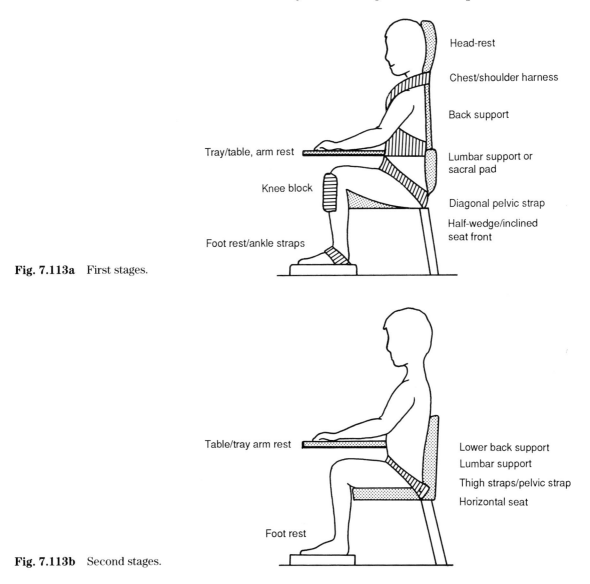

Fig. 7.113a First stages.

Head-rest

Chest/shoulder harness

Back support

Tray/table, arm rest

Lumbar support or sacral pad

Knee block

Diagonal pelvic strap

Half-wedge/inclined seat front

Foot rest/ankle straps

Fig. 7.113b Second stages.

Table/tray arm rest

Lower back support

Lumbar support

Thigh straps/pelvic strap

Horizontal seat

Foot rest

(3) The chair needs to be portable from room to room or transportable for outings. It should not be too cumbersome for homes, classrooms or doorways.

(4) A chair should enable a child to join his family, friends or classmates around a table, on the floor, in a sandpit or at picnics and camps.

(5) A chair does not substitute for therapy and periods of a child's own development of locomotion and postural control.

(6) A child may need more than one chair: one for practising his emerging postural adjustments during looking, listening, reaching

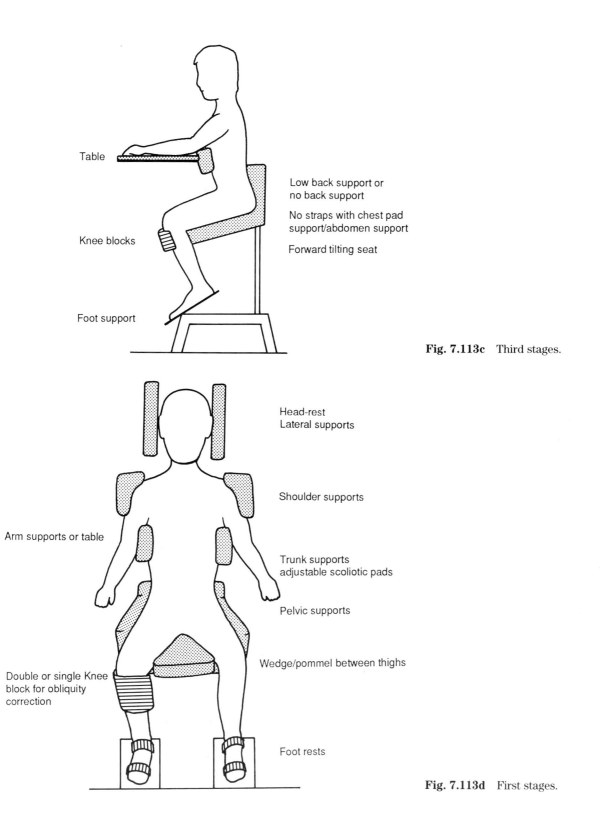

Table

Low back support or
no back support

No straps with chest pad
support/abdomen support

Knee blocks

Forward tilting seat

Foot support

Fig. 7.113c Third stages.

Head-rest
Lateral supports

Shoulder supports

Arm supports or table

Trunk supports
adjustable scoliotic pads

Pelvic supports

Wedge/pommel between thighs

Double or single Knee
block for obliquity
correction

Foot rests

Fig. 7.113d First stages.

out and hand use in all directions; another for safely supporting him during transport and when he is unsupervised and may fall. The additional support maintains postural alignment and stability at times when a child concentrates on difficult communication, visual, hearing and self-care activities. He may have a floor seat and one for a regular table, or, the floor seat can be strapped to a frame at table level with proximity to others at home or at school.

Specific considerations   See Figs 7.98, 7.113, 7.114.

Pelvis, hips and thighs   The position of a child's pelvis is the keystone for better alignment of his head and trunk. It is positioned in association with hips, knees and foot rests. As in postural control training, a child is taught to sit well back in his chair and take weight equally on hips, thighs and feet. When his pelvis is smaller in girth than his trunk, then a sacral

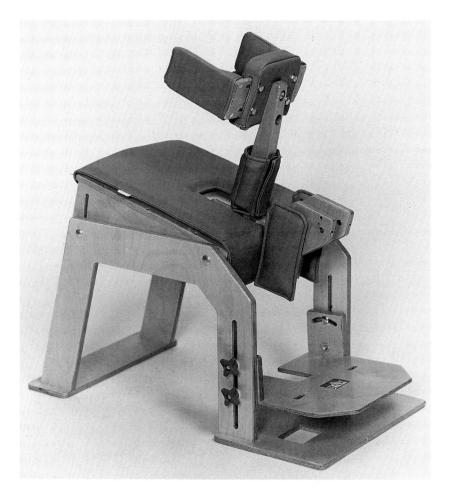

Fig. 7.114 Tilted seat with chest support. Tilt is adjustable and back of child can be observed for symmetry and weight bearing on buttocks. A table can be attached. (With acknowledgements to Jenx for permission.)

pad supports his pelvis as his trunk is supported by the back of his chair. When his body and buttocks change in size then the sacral pad is removed so that protruding buttocks can be accommodated and a lumbar support used. At the same time assessment is made of the developmental stage of a child's pelvic tilt forwards and lumbar mobility. A lumbar support promotes the normal minimal lordosis with vertical pelvic alignment, when a child is at that stage. If not, discomfort and pressure marks are caused.

In order to hold a child's pelvic alignment when he cannot yet do so himself use the following suggestions according to each child.

- A diagonal strap across the front of his hips which ties below the level of his seat to keep hips back against the sacral pad or back of chair.
- A thigh strap for each leg nailed well back between a child's thighs and tying behind and below seat level. Use padding or rubber tubing on the straps to prevent chafing.
- Incline the front of the child's seat (half-wedge) so that his hips flex and his buttocks rest on a flat contoured seat. This prevents a child sliding forward, sacral sitting or hip extensor spasticity. When extensor thrust or tension is severe, then a roll of towel under the knees may help to overcome it by the increased hip flexion. The head and back may also flex as a result and a firm back support with lumbar padding may correct this. If not, try flexing the child's hips with his chest supported in a forward leaning chair with table (Figs 7.113c, 7.114) or against a padded table edge as he stretches his arms forward to grasp bars or lean on forearms.
- Some therapists prevent extensor positions of the hips and sliding out of chairs by tilting the whole chair backwards with the hips flexed between 95° and 110°, as 90° creates forward sliding. This backward tilt has advantages in that it can be a relaxed position for those children who do not have a Moro response, head and trunk thrust in semi-lying or increased athetosis. Backward leaning also fixes the vertebrae in alignment in some cases of scoliosis and in severely involved children with excessive flexion which cannot be straightened otherwise. Most therapists prefer to avoid backward leaning chairs as a child can only see the top of a room, cannot explore visually or locate sounds below him or make face to face contact with children on the floor. Reaching and hand function is more difficult and feeding development needs an upright and slightly flexed head posture. Backward leaning gives a sensation of falling without the proprioception of the vertical posture essential for the development of postural stabilization.
- Knee blocks hold the child's pelvis in position against a sacral pad or back support. They are also used in the forward leaning chair or forward tilted seat for back extension.

- Thigh supports with foot rests may have to be adjusted in relation to the hip flexion used. Take care to avoid pressure behind the knees. Thigh length discrepancies may require shortening of one side of the seat. Observe the position of the knees and check whether pelvic obliquity is the cause of the apparent shortening when knees are not level with each other. Thighs may also straddle a bolster seat (Stewart & McQuilton 1987) in this special design.
- Knee block to correct for pelvic obliquity is needed when this is part of *windswept hips*. A wedge-shaped pommel, thigh or diagonal straps suffice in mild cases. For more severe windsweeping the abducted thigh is pushed back to position the pelvis backwards if it is rotated forwards on that side. The other thigh is abducted as far as possible (Scrutton 1978). If the pelvis is rotated and tipped down on one side then the thigh on that side is flexed on to a small wedge to position the pelvis up and level with the other side. Some severe children benefit from thigh abduction splint alone or when attached to a trunk corset (support) (Fig. 7.115). Trunk posture is then supported and checked for correction of scolioses.
- Lateral pelvis supports and pommels for a wider base also stabilize the pelvis (Fig. 7.113d).

Head and trunk   Once pelvis and hips are aligned then head and trunk are examined further. Add the following if necessary:

- An H harness or shoulder straps to maintain the upright position. A V or crossed harness may be dangerous if a child often drops his head and catches his neck in the harness. Harnesses may be tied behind a child if he enjoys playing and opening the harness buckles.

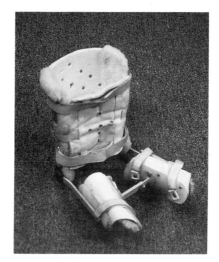

Fig. 7.115

- Lateral chest supports with lateral pelvic supports hold some children in midline if they frequently tip to the side.
- Shoulder supports together with pelvic supports or with trunk supports or even all three supports can hold a child more upright.
- Shoulder supports may be used to bring retracted shoulders forwards so that a severely involved child can reach the table or touch his hands and body.
- The table needs to be adjusted so that kyphoses are corrected and both a child's arms can be used to correct lateral tipping or other asymmetries.
- Hand grasps on correct tray/table heights also assist head and trunk alignment.
- Scoliosis pads are attached to some chairs. The pads need to be moulded to the child's ribs first on the convexity and also on the concavity side at the axilla and at the pelvis.
- Scolioses cannot be corrected by seating on its own and trunk orthoses are necessary. When wearing a corset or other orthosis the child can be upright and the backward tilt of the chair may then be avoided.
- Head control is often activated with adequate trunk and pelvic support with or without a trunk orthosis (see trunk-and-thigh orthosis in Fig. 7.115). Stimulation to hold a child's head up in a chair is usually necessary. However, severely involved children may still benefit from a collar or chin support.
- Usually severely involved children are placed in moulded seats custom made to the shape of their own heads and bodies or to their bodies only (Bardsley, in Eckersley 1993) (Figs 7.116, 7.117).
- Lateral head supports remind children to keep their heads centred, but are unfortunately ineffective in many cases. A child drops his head outside these head blocks in such cases.

Floor seats   Select the correct floor seat so that the young child can play with toys on the floor or join other children playing on the ground in playgroups, playgrounds or sandpits (Figs 7.118–7.120).

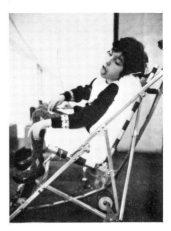

Fig. 7.116

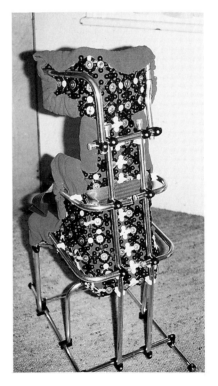

Fig. 7.117

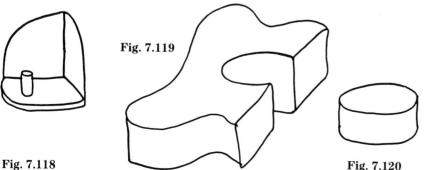

Fig. 7.119

Fig. 7.118

Fig. 7.120

(1) A well padded pommel for adducted legs. Two small pommels may be used close together and gradually moved apart as the child develops more abduction of legs for a wide base.

(2) Height of the back should be at shoulder level of the child if he tends to fall back or arch back when sitting. Occasionally the head may require a padded back support. Curve the chairback to prevent shoulders and back of the child arching into extension. See cylindrical chair (Fig. 7.119).

(3) Height of the back and sides of the floor seat should be cut down to the child's waist level as he acquires more head and trunk control. A square back may be used, as well as triangular and cylindrical ones.

(4) The width of the chair should be such that the child does not slide from side to side. Pad up the sides with sponge or newspapers so that this does not occur. A canvas or inflatable seat allows the child to sink into his own area of support.

(5) Seat of chair is measured from child's hips to his knees.

(6) The floor seat may be placed on wheels for locomotion if the child requires this; it may be used in a toilet seat; it may be tied on to a sturdy adult chair next to the family table. A table can be fitted to it.

(7) The floor seat may have to be raised off the floor for those children who have a very rounded back. The height of the floor seat off the floor should be tested to see whether the child's back straightens. If this does not occur, it is important to give him a table which is high enough for him arms to be elevated to that point where his back straightens. A small firm pillow or back support may help to hold the back straight. Adjusting the position of the pommel (crutch support) may help. If none of these methods corrects a severely rounded back then a *floor seat should not be used.*

OTHER EQUIPMENT FOR SITTING

(1) Chair swings, back and sides on toy trucks, rocking horse or pedal cars. Inflatable chairs, baskets, plastic buckets or bins padded inside and cut out in front, boxes, car seats, cylinder packing cases and various special bath seats and also toilet seats help supported sitting. Children who extend or arch back can be held in sitting using some of this apparatus. However these seats *must* be stabilized near a wall or with weights. They may need a tray, table or low stool at the correct distance from the child so that he can use his hands (Figs 7.121–7.123). *Remember* the child can grasp a horizontal bar to sit.

(2) Toilet seats (Figs 7.124–7.129). See also Chapter 8, Figs 8.1, 8.2.

(3) Push-chairs and wheelchairs (see Appendix).

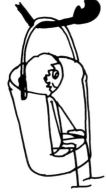

Fig. 7.121 Adapted bucket for sitting.

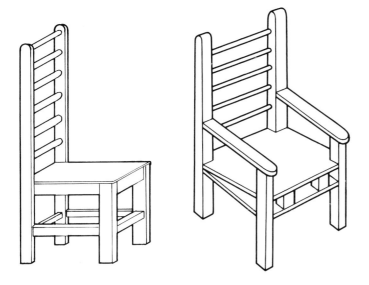

Fig. 7.122 Slatted back based on a design by Petö Institute. Child can sit sideways and hook his arm through slats for balance; use slats to push chair for walking aid. Stabilize base by using a box as base or skis attached. A box base also prevents legs twisting under the seat.

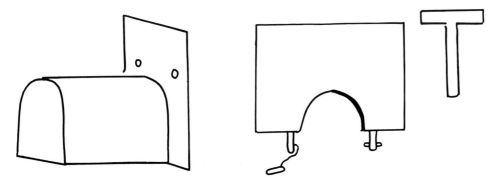

Fig. 7.123 Legs must be abducted over this roll chair (based on a design by Finnie). Knees must be just beneath the top of the roll, and the roll must not be too wide for the child. Check that the child does not slide down one side of the roll. Ordinary low table or fitted cut out table is used. Leave 50 mm (2 inches) between the child's body and the cut out edge.

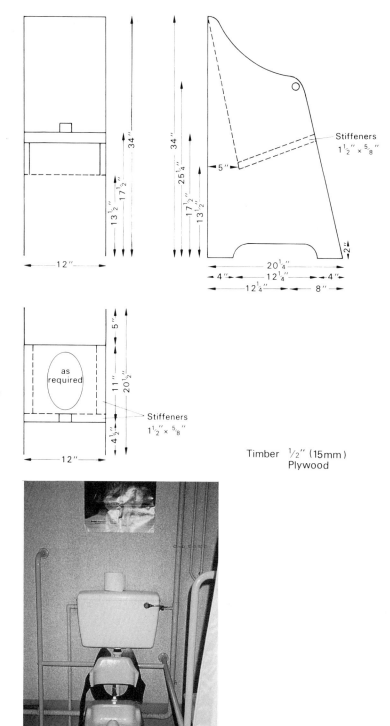

Fig. 7.124 Potty chair, cut hole out to shape of potty. Pad the back and sides of the chair with foam rubber for comfort and cover with a washable fabric. (Scale 1 inch = 25 mm.)

Stiffeners $1\frac{1}{2}$" × $\frac{5}{8}$"

Timber $\frac{1}{2}$" (15 mm) Plywood

Fig. 7.125 Toilet seat.

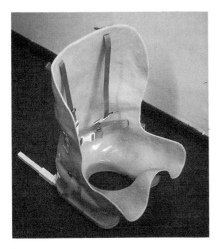

Fig. 7.126 Toilet seat.

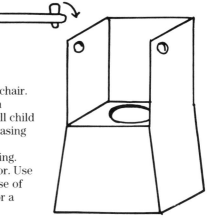

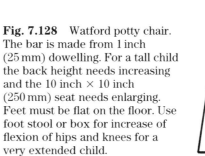

Fig. 7.128 Watford potty chair. The bar is made from 1 inch (25 mm) dowelling. For a tall child the back height needs increasing and the 10 inch × 10 inch (250 mm) seat needs enlarging. Feet must be flat on the floor. Use foot stool or box for increase of flexion of hips and knees for a very extended child.

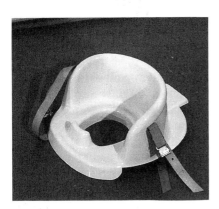

Fig. 7.127 Toilet seat.

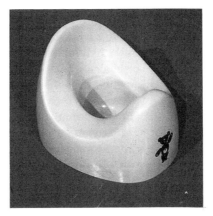

Fig. 7.129 Potty.

Stages in the development of sitting

0–3 Months normal developmental level

COMMON PROBLEMS

Delay in lifting the head up if held fully supported in a sitting position, in holding the head steady. (Head lag in pull-to-sit, see Supine development.)

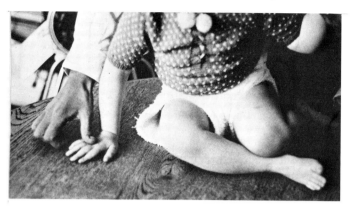

Fig. 7.134 Changing from sitting to side-sitting and back again.

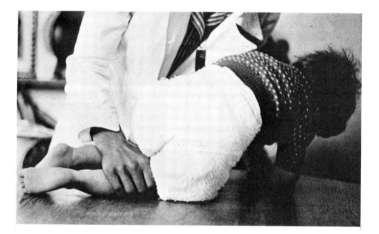

Fig. 7.135 Changing from side-sitting to prone-kneeling (crawl posture) and reverse back again.

The training of various rising patterns seen in normal children may often be corrective for any deformities in children with cerebral palsies. The movements involved activate weight shifts, although *transiently*, rotate the trunk, shoulder and pelvic girdles which result in relaxation of limb spasticity.

(4) Train the child to get on and off low wide stools and then chairs (Fig. 7.136). He often has to use his hands and supports on the seat of the chair or grasp the arm rests, the back of the chair, the table nearby, or hook his arm over the chair or between the rungs of the chairback. Also train the child to get in and out of his wheelchair, in and out of a motor car, toy pedal car, tricycle and other apparatus.

Sitting on a chair and swivelling himself around on the chair is a useful motor ability which is well worth training (Fig. 7.137). Once again the

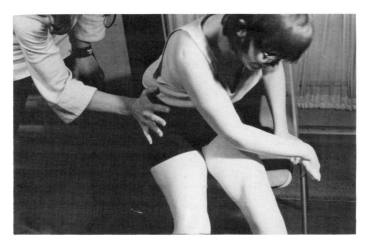

Fig. 7.136 Getting on and off chairs of various heights and widths.

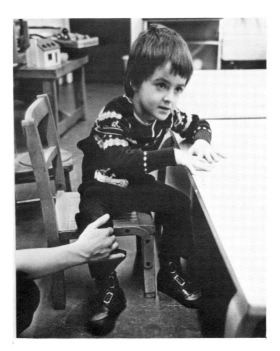

Fig. 7.137 Pivoting on a chair.

postural change is corrective as it teaches separation of adducted legs, trunk control and arm extension, as his hand reaches out for the back of the chair or therapist. Rising from sitting on a chair is now possible and this rising is discussed below.

(5) Practise a variety of sitting postures and reach and grasp in all directions in these postures. Sitting postures include side-sitting

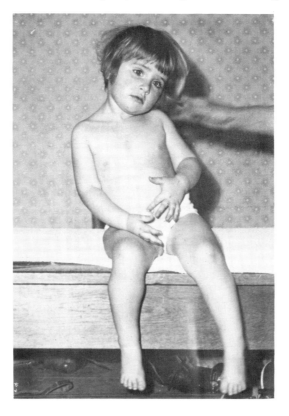

Fig. 7.138 Lateral weight shift stimulated by push off the vertical. A more vigorous push of a child's pelvis/hips well off the horizontal plane stimulates the tilt reaction. If the child falls, saving responses in limbs are activated.

(Fig. 7.134), sitting with one foot flat on the ground the other bent or straight, sitting with both knees bent and feet flat on the ground (crook-sitting), sitting in various types of chairs of the correct size and in adult chairs if the child is correctly placed.

(6) Augment sitting with manual resistance given laterally, with rotation, anteroposteriorly (Fig. 7.111).

(7) Postural adjustment and weight shift as well as tilt reactions and saving reactions in the limbs are all stimulated by slow and by quick pushes (Fig. 7.138). Use rocking chairs, rocking horses, swings, see-saws, rocker boat or toys, and inflatable toys to help develop the tilt reactions and security in sitting. Play 'see-saw' games on parent's lap or body. Pony riding and horse riding stimulate tilt (Fig. 7.139).

DEVELOPMENT OF STANDING AND WALKING

The following main aspects should be developed:

Antigravity support or weight bearing on feet. Normally present at birth and modified at 6 months.

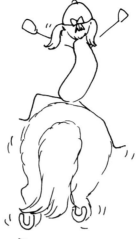

Fig. 7.139

Postural fixation of the head on the trunk (Fig. 7.140) and on the pelvis in the vertical. Normally present by 9–12 months (see sitting).

Postural fixation of the pelvic girdle in the vertical. Normally present by 9–12 months (see upright kneeling supported, and supported standing).

Counterpoising in the standing position when holding on (Fig. 7.141), i.e. normally at 9–12 months level, and without holding on, 12–18 months, becoming more varied in the second and third year of life. Examples are: lifting an arm or standing on one foot, holding on at 9–11 months

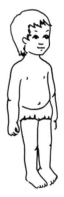

Fig. 7.140 Postural fixation, head on trunk on pelvis and whole of child in standing.

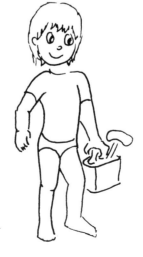

Fig. 7.141 Counterpoising a weight or movement of the arm.

normally and much later on one foot, and not holding on, at 2½–3 years of age normally. Standing on one foot is a most important counterpoising reaction. The child can then take weight on one leg for long enough to allow the other to swing through and step. Prepare for one foot balance by weight shift from side to side.

Control of antero-posterior weight shift of the child's centre of gravity to initiate walking (propulsion) and to stop (retropulsion). Later in a diagonal direction and in turning (12–24 months normally).

Control of lateral sway from one foot to the other. Normally developed in cruising and walking each hand held laterally, and similar activities about 12 months of age. Lateral sway is very obvious in toddlers and becomes modified with development.

Tilt reactions in standing are anteroposterior and lateral. They are acquired after standing and walking alone. Tilt reactions are not important for standing and walking. However, children without tilt reactions will be unsure in the dark and on rough ground.

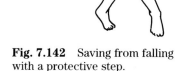

Fig. 7.142 Saving from falling with a protective step.

Saving from falling (Fig. 7.142)   If tilt reactions fail the child will take a protective step out to save himself (staggering). He also flings out his arms in protective (saving) reactions. Normally these develop at 12–24 months of age. They are important as the child will have less fear of falling if he can protect himself, and may then become willing to walk.

Foley (personal communication) has described various abnormalities of gait associated with the absence of one or more of the above mechanisms. These problems are treated in the practical suggestions below.

Rising reactions (7.143) from lying (prone and supine) to standing, from sitting to standing and from kneeling to standing. Some have already been discussed in the sections on supine, sitting and prone development. (See also Fig. 7.184.)

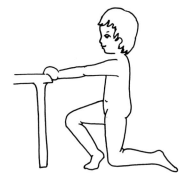

Fig. 7.143   Rising to standing.

Note If a child cannot stand up, or rise and get up to standing, he may *still be able* to stand and walk. However he will depend on someone to place him in standing, and if this is not done standing and walking may be retarded for this reason.

Stages in the development of standing and walking (Figs 7.144–7.155)

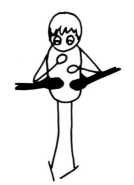

Fig. 7.144 Weight bearing on legs (supporting reaction) (*0–3 months*).

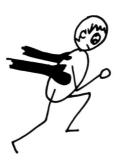

Fig. 7.145 Automatic stepping if infant is tilted forward (*0–3 months*).

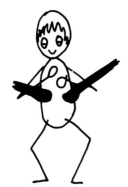

Fig. 7.146 Sinking or astasia (*3–6 months*). Head control.

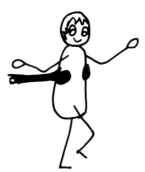

Fig. 7.147 Trunk supported standing and bouncing in standing (*5–7 months*).

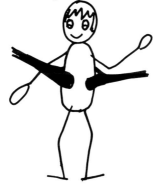

Fig. 7.148 Supported standing (*5–7 months*).

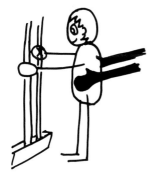

Fig. 7.149 Stand holding on to support with pelvic support (*7–9 months*).

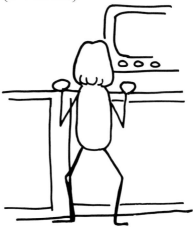

Fig. 7.150 Stand holding on to furniture (*7–9 months*). Begin weight shift.

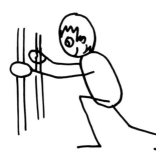

Fig. 7.151 Pull up to standing from various positions (*9–12 months*).

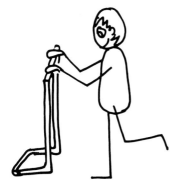

Fig. 7.152 Stand holding and lift one leg off the ground (*11 months*).

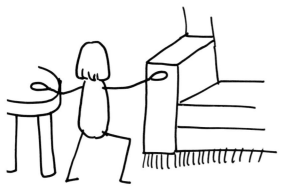

Fig. 7.153 Cruising (lateral stepping) (*9–12 months*).

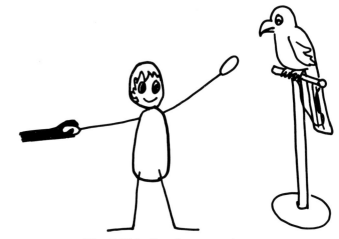

Fig. 7.154 Stand supported, reach in all directions (*9–12 months*). Weight shift.

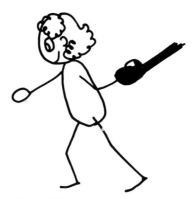

Fig. 7.155 Stand alone and walk with two hands, then one, then no hand support (*12–18 months*).

Abnormal postures in standing (see also Figs 7.170–7.175).

These may be due to:

Absence of postural fixation The child may be able to maintain equilibrium, even inadequately, by attempting an abnormal posture to compensate for this absence (Fig. 7.156). He may be:

(1) *Sinking* into hip flexion, knee flexion, with or without:
(2) Adduction-internal rotation of the legs.

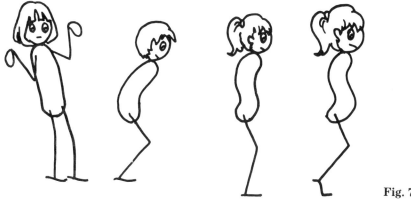

Fig. 7.156

(3) Lordosis may compensate for hip flexion.
(4) Round back and head flexion may be present.
(5) Feet in valgus or in overdorsiflexion. If overdorsiflexion is limited by tightness of ankle or plantarflexors, the child may stand on his toes.

Alternatively the child may fall or extend backwards and compensate by (Figs 7.157, 7.158):

(1) Hip flexion.
(2) Hyperextension of knees.
(3) Internal rotation of legs, occasionally
(4) Valgus feet or normal feet.
(5) Rounding his back and jutting his head forward.

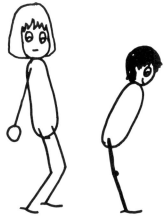

Fig. 7.157

These postures, to maintain equilibrium under difficult circumstances, are also seen in normal people on slippery surfaces or when first attempting ice skating or skiing.

If the child also has spasticity or rigidity he may use that to prop himself up (see below). Spastic muscles shorten and maintain the abnormal postures above. They may create abnormal postures in some children due to the biomechanical effect of shortened muscles and tendons.

If the child has *good* upper limbs or at least a grasp in poor upper limbs, he will use them for support. Such children *stand and walk on their hands* with walking aids (Fig. 7.159). They bear so much weight on their hands that fatigue of the good arms is common. Athetoid children are known to hold their shoulders and arms forward and together to stop the backward fall.

Fear of falling is naturally appropriate when postural control is so inadequate. Fears exacerbate all these abnormal postures.

be left with straight legs but completely loses his independent standing or even stumbling around.

Some athetoid children have been observed to use an asymmetrical tonic neck reaction. The face turning to one side increases hypertonus in the weight bearing leg on that side, so that they can then bear weight on it.

It is interesting that some workers call children with spasticity 'children with too much fixation' meaning postural fixation, and call children with rigidity 'children with too much postural stability' (Goff 1969). It is that they have *no* or poor normal postural fixation or stability and use hypertonicity to prop them up against gravity.

Biomechanics and spasticity   Spasticity may be greater in one group than another. If a resulting deformity is greater in one joint it leads to abnormal postures in the others to maintain a fairly upright position. These postures may also become deformities. For example:

(1)   Hip flexion may be dictated by greater knee flexion.
(2)   Hip flexion may be dictated by equinus in order not to extend and fall back.
(3)   Knee flexion may be dictated by too much hip flexion to avoid falling forward.
(4)   Hip flexion-adduction-internal rotation may be dictated by valgus flexed knees.
(5)   Hip extension may occur by hamstrings flexing the knees and tilting the pelvis backwards. A long kyphosis or a flat back may be associated.
(6)   Knee flexion or knee hyperextension may compensate for tight plantarflexors or equinus.
(7)   Equinus may be secondary to excessive hip and knee flexion and the spastic plantarflexors cannot remain stretched by the mechanical overdorsiflexion.
(8)   Lordosis compensates for hip flexion.
(9)   Kypholordosis compensates for hip flexion.

Clearly abnormal postures or deformities are rarely localized in one joint. Thus one spastic muscle group with its weak antagonists should never be considered alone in treatment, with or without orthopaedic surgery.

The spastic child's abnormal posture may be different when he has to maintain his balance on his own. Thus abnormal postures are:

Supported standing
●   Hip extension or semiflexion, adduction with legs together or crossing (scissoring), internal rotation.
●   Knee extension.
●   Equinus or *on toes*.

Later in unsupported standing
- Hip flexion, adduction-internal rotation.
- Knee flexion or hyperextension or normal.
- Feet equinovarus, varus (supination), valgus (pronation), sometimes heel may be down and forefoot everted.
- Toes may clench and evert.
- Lordosis, kyphosis, flattening of lumbar area or kypholordosis.
- Pelvic tilt backwards is associated with flat back, pelvic tilt forwards with lordosis.

Perturbations of a child in standing   Nashner *et al.* (1983) have shown in their studies that the sequence of muscle activation in a cerebral palsied child differs from that of an able-bodied child. Nevertheless, such a child with cerebral palsy does not fall over.

ARM AND HEAD POSTURES

These are similar to the abnormal postures seen in the lower levels of the child's development. However, if the hands are grasped by an adult or the child holds on for support he may use an abnormal pattern in arms and hands. The spastic child usually increases flexion-adduction in shoulder, shoulder hunching, flexion-pronation in elbow, palmar flexion with or without ulnar deviation in hands, adduction of thumbs. Increase in flexion in the arms often seems to increase flexion in the legs and aggravate the abnormal postures of the whole child, and vice versa. Increase of abnormal shoulder extension often associates with hip extension. Athetoids who abduct and hold their arms up abnormally with elbows flexed, also tend to grasp supports abnormally and aggravate their backward fall or lean. The child may flex his head or *poke* his chin forward in standing.

Abnormal gait

The problems in standing will affect the gait, therefore walking should not be 'pushed' if standing is absent or very abnormal. Fears of falling may increase abnormal gait patterns in such cases.

Delay or abnormal walking patterns may be due to:

Poor or absent fixation and counterpoising or asymmetrical ability to counterpoise   The child may *waddle* from side to side without counterpoising each leg, that is he 'falls' from foot to foot as he cannot maintain posture for any length of time on one side. There may be excessive trunk sway from side to side. The pelvis and trunk may rotate forward on the side of the swing-through (stepping) leg instead of counterpoising on to the weight bearing leg in an upright position. The child may have a better postural mechanism on one side, most obviously seen in hemiplegia or asymmetrical quadriplegias or triplegias (asymmetrical ability). A limp on to the good side is then characteristic of the gait.

Athetoid children may *run headlong* as they cannot bear weight long enough on each side for a step. Athetoid children and ataxic children stumble about for this and other reasons. Cerebral palsied children, children with intellectual impairment and others who are only motor delayed, will not wish to walk, show fear of walking and hang on to adults excessively and on to their walking aids. Excessive arm flinging movements or emphasis of the saving reactions in the arms come into play to help the child balance on each unstable leg. 'Sinking' patterns of standing and compensation for falling back are seen as in standing (see Figs 7.156–7.159).

Absence of anteroposterior shift   This makes it impossible for the child to *start* walking. A walking aid on wheels may start him off. Stopping is also difficult if this mechanism is not operating. He may also *mark time* and then stop, as he is unable to stop or reverse the anteroposterior shift. Some children only stop by a collapse onto their bottoms.

Absence of lateral sway   This is obvious in the athetoid running headlong and other children pushing wheelwalkers. In treatment, lateral sway is helped by training standing on one foot (counterpoising), and is also developed in cruising sideways and other activities.

Lack of tilt reactions in prone, supine, sitting, upright kneel and standing rarely delays walking. This training in walking should not be delayed if these reactions are not yet acquired. Martin (1967) found that labyrinthectomized adults could walk although tilt reactions were not possible without their labyrinths. Similar observations have been noted in children who walk but have absent or poor tilt reactions. Nevertheless, tilt reactions should be included in the programme as it makes the child more steady in changes of terrain and in the dark. As Dr Foley puts it 'you cannot walk across a ploughed field at night if you do not have tilt reactions' (personal communication).

Saving or protective reaction (arms and legs)   These must be trained to prevent the danger of the child falling on his face, and giving him confidence to walk. Remember that the protective step in falling is not the same as a voluntary step which the child takes as he is being trained to walk. Foley observed the presence of voluntary stepping without the presence of protective stepping and vice versa (personal communication). Therapy must therefore train both of those stepping movements. Excessive saving reactions in arms or legs may occur to compensate for the absence of the other mechanisms. It is most noticeable in ataxic children and athetoid children. The *drunken walk* may be excessive staggering reactions in the legs. Athetoid children cannot *stand still* but take little protective steps.

Forssberg (1985) and Leonard *et al.* (1988, 1991), among others, have contributed studies on abnormal gait patterns compared to normal children's walking.

SPASTIC GAITS

All the problems above will be included with the addition of the pull of spasticity and associated weakness. There may be abnormal postures which are associated with each other, as described in the section on Abnormal postures in standing.

HIPS AND KNEES

Hips may adduct and cross when the child is supported, and adduct-internally rotate and flex when the child is walking independently. Flexion occurs as the leg is swinging through and/or on weight bearing (stance).

Knees may overflex on swing through and on weight bearing. Hip and knee flexion may occur to allow a plantarflexed foot (or toe pointing foot) to swing and clear the ground, and once on the ground hip and knee flexion occur to push the heel to the ground. *Toe first* and not the normal heel strike is common in spastics.

Lack of heel strike after swing through may be compensated differently.

In hemiplegia and other spastics the hip alone may flex with hyper-extension of the knee to press the heel to the ground. This is usual with extensor spasticity or excessive antigravity support as the forefoot strikes the ground.

A wide base is used with flexed adducted (valgus) knees as the spastic child cannot balance on the small base created by adduction of the hips.

FEET

Walking on the toes is seen if the child is supported and later when he walks alone. There is not only weight bearing on the toes but the toes are brought down first for weight bearing (see above).

Walking on the toes may become walking on a pronated-everted (valgus) foot in the child's efforts to compensate for spastic plantarflexors.

Walking on toes may be accompanied by slightly flexed hips and even straight knees or slightly flexed in younger or milder cases.

A rare *normal ballerina walk* has been observed (Holt 1973). Hips and knees are straight and flexibe. I have also observed this in toddlers with severe visual impairment without any cerebral palsy.

PELVIS AND TRUNK

The pelvis often rotates abnormally in spastic gaits. The rotation may be backwards so the leg appears *retracted* and behind the other. Usually the front, better leg may take more weight, as in hemiplegia. However the back leg may take more weight and allow the forward leg to step, take its momentary weight and then transfer on to the back leg, which only has time to take a small step and *cannot* get in front of the forward leg.

Pelvic tilt is also backwards with flattening of the lumbar area, or pelvic tilt forwards with a lordosis of the lumbar area. Kyphosis of the thorax may occur with flat back or lordosis. Scoliosis may be present due to unequal weight distribution, leg length and other reasons already given for asymmetry in standing and sitting.

If the child takes a step, his spasticity may be so great that he has to lean back to push his leg forward. He has an anteroposterior *waddle* or jerky walk. Lateral waddle is associated with spastic adductors and weak abductors. It is also involved with inability to fixate the pelvis when counterpoising in standing on one leg. The trunk and head may lean forward to help overcome spasticity as well as maintain balance (see above). This usually *increases* toe walking as the child cannot put his heels down in this pattern.

ARMS

Excessive arm swing up, arms held up in the air, or excessive saving reactions may occur in the arms. Therefore, normal reciprocal arm swing may be absent. Abnormal postures of arms may be seen as in earlier motor developmental skills. The retraction of the shoulder may accompany retraction of the pelvis and hip. See Figs 7.170–7.179. Some athetoid movements of a child's arms may throw him off balance.

SUMMARY

Abnormal features of gait for therapy
Excessive (1)   Hip and trunk sway from side to side or a pelvic waddle.
       (2)   Hip and trunk sway anteroposterior and jerky gait.
       (3)   Asymmetry of weight bearing and unequal steps.
       (4)   Abnormal postures of head, trunk, pelvis, knees and feet.
       (5)   Abnormal stepping patterns, e.g. walk on toes.
       (6)   Athetoid *running gait*; *drunken gait* of ataxics or athetoids; *high stepping gait* or *scissoring gait* in spastics or athetoids.
       (7)   Overactive arms to maintain balance, *tightrope walking* or abnormal arm postures and lack of reciprocal arm swing.

Treatment suggestions at all levels of development

PRACTICAL POINTS

Train standing (fixation and counterpoising) and postural alignment *first*, *and also* when child is walking independently, but with an abnormal gait. All the abnormal gaits discussed above will be treated in a programme concentrating on:

(1) Equal distribution of weight on each foot.
(2) Correction of abnormal postures.
(3) Building up of the child's stability by decreasing support.
(4) Delay training in standing and walking if the child is not ready.
(5) Continuing to develop head, trunk and pelvic postural fixation and counterpoising in sitting, support 'on hands' in upright kneeling, half-kneeling and in vertical positions other than standing, as well as in standing.
(6) Weight shift leading to stepping.
(7) Training lateral sway and cruising and walk holding support each side.
(8) Training stopping and starting and turning and walking on uneven ground, and using stairs and inclines.

(1) Equal distribution of weight bearing on each foot   Supported and later unsupported standing
(a) Check this by having child standing on two weighing scales and help him correct this as you read the *equal* weight borne on each scale.
(b) Head and trunk in midline supported and then unsupported after 9 month level of normal development.
(c) Teach weight shift cn to the side that bears less weight. Do this by asking and assisting the child to move himself on to the leg. If possible, ask the child to move against your hand placed firmly against his lateral hip.
(d) Use a mirror for both you and the child to see that he is in correct alignment with his weight on both feet.
(e) Use a wide base and then bring both feet together for standing, then move one foot in front of the other.
(f) Correct any deformities, especially of the feet, such as equinus, so that there are *two* plantigrade feet for equal weight bearing. Equinus may be secondary to other deformities, see below.
(g) Check length of legs in case of growth asymmetries and raise shoe if there is more than $\frac{1}{2}$-inch (12.5 mm) difference.
(h) Remember to keep the child's weight forward over both feet and not allow him to twist or lean backwards. Do *not* let him *lean back* against the wall, standing apparatus or an adult.

(i)   Whenever possible face a child. He uses your presence as motivation to stand in correct postural alignment with gravity.

(2)   Correct abnormal postures or deformities
See correction of abnormal postures in sitting and use the same methods for kyphosis, scoliosis, hip adduction and internal rotation, feet deformities.

(a)   Place the child's legs apart in standing, hips and knees turned outward with head and back upright, knees straight and feet flat on the ground, facing outwards. Stand him like this over a roll of blankets, inflatable toy, sponge rubber, large stuffed toy or wide toy truck. You can hold him like this when you are seated on the floor and the child's legs are abducted over your thigh or legs. Hold the child's knees and thighs facing apart and outward (in external rotation). The toy he straddles may have to keep his *knees and feet* apart. Press his heels to the ground by pushing down through his knees to his heels.

(b)   Equal weight distribution and weight forward over feet will correct many abnormal postures. Symmetrical postures and head in midline corrects asymmetry. Motivate and facilitate child's arm reach overhead to overcome a rounded back or bent hips and knees (Figs 7.109, 7.170).

(c)   In all methods keep a child's arms either in symmetrical extension at his sides; or at right angles at his shoulders, over a roll or on a couch; or with the weight of the child taken through his elbows or through his hands; or with the child grasping a bar in front of him with his *elbows extended* or bars at each side of him, or broomsticks, with elbows extended. The child keeps his head in the centre and his back as straight as possible (Figs 7.160–7.165).

(d)   Splints and braces. If abnormal positions cannot be actively corrected by the child *in every joint*, at the same time, splintage or bracing should be used for one joint whilst the others are actively corrected by him. For example, correct abnormal adduction with abduction pants or an abduction splint, whilst training the child to stretch his knees and keep his heels down with his weight taken towards the external surface of his feet. Another possibility is to correct bent knees with the knee corsets, or polythene knee pieces, whilst the child actively corrects the position of hips and feet. Yet another possibility is to correct the feet in below-knee irons or in plaster-of-Paris whilst the child actively corrects hips and knees, head and trunk.

Orthopaedic surgery in selected cases having hip flexion-adduction-internal rotation, knee flexion and equinus, equinovarus or equinovalgus and postoperative physiotherapy (Sharrard 1971; Samilson 1975; Bleck 1987).

(3)   Building up child's own stability by a decrease of
support given to him
Carry out methods with trunk or shoulders supported by your hands, standing frame or standing box. Then hold the child supported at his waist, then hips, then thighs and knees. This is equivalent to developmental levels 0–9 months. At 9–11 months his own hand grasp is spontaneously used for support, but before this, the child's hands will have to be placed on to bars for grasp. Hold his hands on a bar by gently pressing down on his wrists. To overcome any fears let a child tell a therapist when she should 'let go' so that he can balance with less or no support.

Note: weight bearing and stepping are not walking   Children who are able to bear weight and reflex step without trunk balance are really at 0–6 months normal developmental level. These children are frequently the ones who support themselves under their arms in walking frames on wheels and run headlong in them. Some athetoid children who run headlong, but are unable to stand alone, are mostly at this developmental level, having not yet developed the postural fixation of head, trunk and pelvis of later trimesters. Some ataxic children can also bear weight and step in walkers. If there are wheels on the walkers, they will stagger in all directions. The training of standing and walking in such children, including athetoid children and ataxic children, should concentrate on the next trimesters of development which build up trunk and pelvic control.

(4)   Delay the training of standing and walking
in the following instances:
(a)   Abnormal weight bearing, without the trunk and pelvic control of later (3–9 months) levels of development may be particularly severe. If excessive antigravity reaction of hip adduction (scissoring) internal rotation, hip and knee extension, toe standing occurs when the child is held in standing and this reaction cannot be corrected, or only corrected with difficulty, by the therapist, then the training of standing should be *delayed*. This is frequently a problem with spastic children. Treatment in these cases should concentrate on prone, supine and sitting development. An inclined *prone stander* with control of feet, knees and hips with an abduction wedge (pommel) may be appropriate so that a child can be placed at eye level with his peers who are standing. This incline is adjusted to avoid excessive antigravity reactions.
(b)   Delay standing and walking in the case when the excessive antigravity reaction (supporting reaction) is only controlled at the cost

of *abnormal overflow*. The reaction can be controlled and corrected manually or by equipment, so that the legs are kept apart, knees straight facing out and heels down. However, the leg postures may be correct *but* at the cost of an increase of hypertonus in the arms and hands, or trunk. Check whether this *overflow* can be corrected at once. If not, although the development of standing may proceed, there will be a loss or decrease of hand function or increase of deformity in the upper limbs and trunk. Thus, treatment suggestions for standing should be followed when the child is more ready to respond to them. This will be after a period of training the pelvic and trunk fixation mechanisms in prone, supine and sitting development and occasionally in upright kneeling. Development of these postural mechanisms does seem to decrease excessive hypertonus during weight bearing on the feet when these children are finally placed in standing.

(5)   Continue training of head, trunk and pelvic control in other developmental levels during training of standing
Train this control in sitting, knee walking (sideways, forward, backward), half kneeling and upright kneeling, and emphasize postural fixation and counterpoising mechanisms. *Do not use upright kneeling* if the child has hip or knee flexion tightness or lordosis. Even if the older child is walking, these mechanisms may still have to be trained, to *improve* his pattern of walking (gait). See 0–12 months developmental levels below, for these mechanisms in standing development.

Points (6), (7) and (8) above are discussed in the developmental level 9–12 months, below, as well as in later development.

Stages in the development of standing and walking

0–3 Months normal developmental level

COMMON PROBLEMS

Delay in taking weight on feet, when supported on soles.

Abnormal performance   See Abnormal postures in standing, supported.

Reflex reactions
(1)   Excessive antigravity response, see Abnormal postures in standing.
(2)   Persistence of automatic stepping after 1–2 months.
(3)   Various abnormal stepping reactions such as *athetoid dance*, when each leg withdraws outwards with eversion on sole contact with the ground. Sole contact may also include grasping reflex of the ground.

Some athetoids 'conflict between grasp and withdrawal reflexes' (Twitchell 1961), in one leg only a *pawing* repetitive involuntary motion of this leg.

(4) Excessive *crossed extension reflex* seen in a jerky high stepping pattern, with the other leg rigidly extended as its sole contacts the ground. This is similar to automatic stepping above.

(5) Withdrawal reflex of both feet on contact with the ground, as opposed to alternate withdrawals of each leg.

TREATMENT SUGGESTIONS AND DAILY CARE

Increase weight bearing on both feet which counteracts delay as well as the various abnormal reactions to foot contact with floor. Trunk support is needed at this stage.

(1) Use of knee gaiters, polythene knee-splints, long leg irons or braces (Appendix).

(2) Periods of weight bearing in apparatus, e.g. frames, standing boxes or cut out tables (Fig. 7.160).

(3) Joint compression through hips and pelvis or through knees (Fig. 7.161).

(4) Desensitize soles of feet by weight bearing on feet with heels pressed down in sitting, squatting and in standing. Use shoes and various floor surfaces, sponge or a trampoline etc. to find which the child can tolerate. Inclined *prone stander* allows partial pressure of child's weight on his feet and aids such toleration (Fig. 7.160).

(5) Prone standers are used to correct postures of trunk and legs. Select elements for each child. Prone standers do not train postural stabilization for standing as do upright frames.

Correct abnormal postures within methods in Figs 7.160, 7.161.

Note   Give full trunk support for use of methods at this level (Fig. 7.160).

Prone standers or inclined frames do not train standing itself, but correct postures and desensitize soles of feet. Upright positions are needed to train standing (later stages).

3–5 Months normal developmental level

This is the level at which the normal baby does not take weight in standing but sags (astasia). The next level of development should be attempted from time to time until there is a flicker of response, then work at 6–9 months level on the development of standing.

Fig. 7.160a,b,c,d Child's arms symmetrical, head and trunk central, weight equal on each foot. Keep child's weight forward on to his feet. Trunk is supported by a roll, a large ball, table, high couch or the body of the therapist behind him. Also use a high couch, ledges on an ordinary table with padded edge, rounded edge or cut-out table. Later remove the trunk support and use his hand grasp on support, or lean only on forearms, lean on hands on low table (9–12 months level) and then higher tables. Legs are apart and externally rotated, hips flexed or extended, knees straight, feet flat on the ground. Use orthosis or abduction pants, knee corsets, foot supports according to the child's difficulties. To assume corrected position use methods in Figs 7.180–7.184. Rhythmically shift the knees into semiflexion to avoid rigid infantile stance. Hold his knees to do this, especially if the knees also hyperextend. Later shift weight from foot to foot (see Fig. 7.163). (d) Prone stander. Height and angle are adjusted so that pelvis is aligned without hyperextension of back or head. Lateral adjustment of pelvic band with derotation and adjustment of knee blocks obtains symmetrical weight bearing. Incorporate foot block if legs are of different lengths. Table is adjusted for hand function and for head control with chin in. Table may be angled or horizontal. Time in any stander needs supervision so that excessive use does not increase hypertonus or fatigue (30–60 minutes). (With acknowledgement to James Leckey Design, Dunmurry, Northern Ireland.)

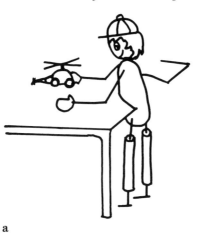

a

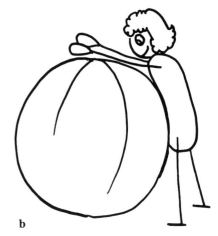

b

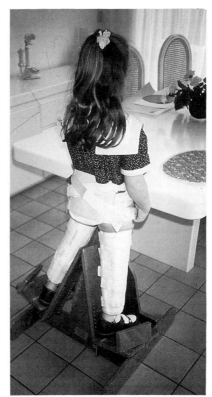

c

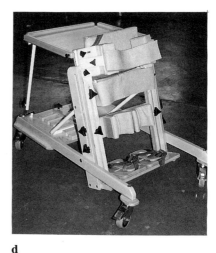

d

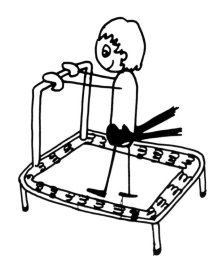

Fig. 7.161 Joint compression through hips, later through knees. Child may stand on floor, but trampoline, sponge rubber, inflatable mattress may be used if posture is kept corrected, and *bouncing is restricted*. The trunk may be supported by his own grasp or holding your shoulders (9–12 months level) or if his trunk requires more support (6–9 months level) lean child against table, roll, couch, large stuffed stable toy, or large ball. Head and body alignment must be well over straight legs and feet on the ground. Avoid hyperextension of knees and any abnormal postures as in Figs 7.156–7.159.

6–9 Months normal developmental level

COMMON PROBLEMS

Delay in weight bearing with flexible knees, if supported, active *bounce* when held in standing, alternate stepping (not automatic high stepping), if held with hip flexion, knee extension and heels down on the floor and beginning to stand alone grasping a support.

Abnormal performance See abnormal posture in standing, supported, above.

Reflex reactions Those expected to develop at this level are:

(1) Parachute or saving reactions in the arms on falling forward or sideways (see Development of sitting, Figs 7.79 and 7.138).
(2) Propping reactions in the arms to *break* the fall (see sitting, Fig. 7.87).
(3) Tilt reactions in sitting which may make standing more secure if not directly related to its acquisition.
(4) Presence of toe clenching in supported standing until about 9 months level.
(5) Persistence of reflex reactions from 0–3 months is abnormal.

PHYSIOTHERAPY SUGGESTIONS AND DAILY CARE

See Figs 7.160, 7.161 and Appendix Fig. 2.

9–12 Months normal developmental level

COMMON PROBLEMS

Delay in standing, holding on and releasing one hand, releasing one leg to stand on the other, stepping sideways or cruising. Inability to stand alone momentarily, step two-handed support, one-handed support. Delay in rise from prone or supine to standing with help given in the transitional positions of either sitting, kneeling on all fours and half-kneeling. Delay in pulling himself to standing from kneeling holding on, from sitting or from hands and knees.

Abnormal performance of standing posture, see abnormal posture in standing, supported and unsupported (above); abnormal gait, above.

Reflex reactions   Those expected at this level are the saving reactions in the arms if falling backwards as well as propping on hands to break the fall (see Development of sitting, Figs 7.79 and 7.138).

PHYSIOTHERAPY SUGGESTIONS

Remove support from child's trunk, and later from pelvis.

Improve stability with the following techniques: the child stands, holding on or alone. Apply manual pressure at his hips or shoulders pushing him off balance, he must actively maintain his upright standing – 'Don't let me push you over'. Do this laterally and also anteroposteriorly (Fig. 7.162). Do this with rotation – 'Don't let me turn you'. Another way of using resistance is to ask the child to push against your hands placed in positions on his hips or shoulders or on one hip and one shoulder – 'Push against my hands'. Resistance should not be *so great* that the child twists his limbs into abnormal positions, or increases involuntary movements, or even falls over!

Stand and sway (Figs 7.162–7.164)   Train lateral sway with legs apart then together. At first the child is swayed from side to side, then shifts his weight along or against your hand on his hip, shoulder, or hip and shoulder. Augment weight shift against your hand offering resistance. Carry this out initially with support to child's chest or having him lean on his forearms, on hands, or grasping a support with elbows straight.

   Child's grasp should be forward, sideways at waist and at shoulder level. Lateral grasp on poles is preferable to parallel bars as it improves symmetrical weight bearing, back and head position and trains supinated grasp. Release grasp as soon as control is possible without it. Lateral sway prepares child for cruising and is part of good gait training. Use this action as child reaches out for toys.

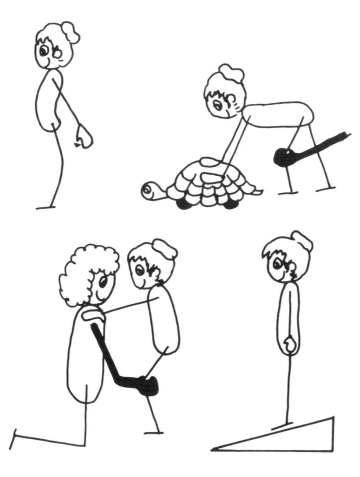

Fig. 7.175 Correction of hyperextended knees and lordosis.

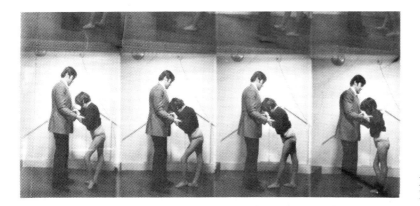

Fig. 7.176 Hyperextended knees.

rings lightly held in each of your hands or both of you hold on to a large ball (netball size) simultaneously as you step. Always ensure that his weight is well forward over his base.

(3) Walk holding someone's hands on either side or in front of him.

(4) Walk pushing a weighted doll's pram, another child in his wheel-chair, a child's chair, a kitchen chair, a chair on wooden skis or with set of runners, or a metal walker on four points which slide (Appendix).

(5) Walking using crutches, elbow crutches, tripods, quadripods or sticks.

(6) Walking using vertical poles at either side with thick rubber bases (Fig. 7.171).

When using walking aids consider the following

Grasping a support at the side of the child tends to train lateral sway for walking. However, if the support involves elbow flexion this may be contraindicated in spastics as the grasp-elbow flexion and hunching of the shoulders increases spasticity in the arms and may also overflow into the legs. The child's grasps need to be low down and slightly in front with straight elbows (Figs 7.177–7.179). Use elbow gaiters to assist extension. You may instead hold both his elbows straight as you bring his weight within and slightly in front of his base.

Grasping the hand support in front helps to train the anteroposterior

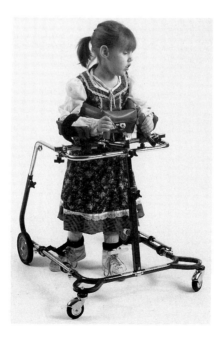

Fig. 7.177   Walker for child needing chest support and forward lean. Forearms can be adjusted further forward. Forearm support assists symmetrical shoulder stability and grasp in midposition. Select walkers such as Cheyne walker, Arrow walker and others for elbow extension in children who habitually flex elbows and also require forward lean and chest support. (Acknowledgement to Rifton for this Rifton Gait trainer.)

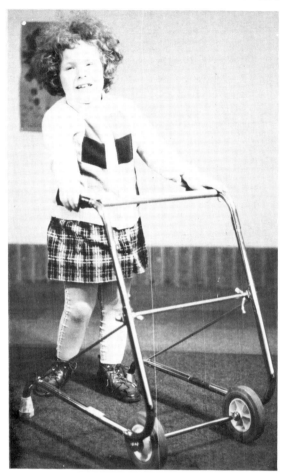

Fig. 7.178 Rollator.

shift needed to start walking. Once again show or use elbow gaiters for straight elbows. It may also be helpful to press a child's wrists down to improve his grasp. Try having him lean forward and down on to open hands or forward onto his grasp. This is most effective in training the initiation of stepping and continuation of stepping. In Fig. 7.174, note the open hands of the therapist allowing the child to press down and forward to initiate stepping.

Inadequate hand use for walking aids Some athetoid movements interfere with a child's maintenance of grasp. Children with severe intellectual disabilities or perceptual problems may not manage to use walking aids as well as concentrate on balance and stepping. Hold these children's hands on to the bars directly or by pressing through their wrists as they grasp. Use particularly stable walking frames, weighted trolleys or doll's prams. The ladderback chair or chair on padded wooden skis is often

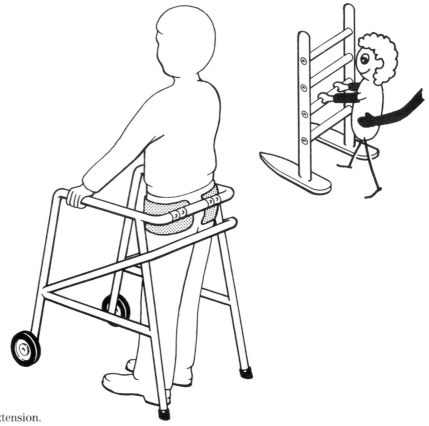

Fig. 7.179   Walkers to promote extension.

helpful. Avoid walkers with castors or wheels, which run too quickly for a child. Later crutches with weighted bases may be managed by some children.

Baby walkers or walkers with a body ring and canvas sling or seat with castors. These mass-produced walkers are not usually safe for any baby as they tip over easily. The wheels on all four corners create undesirable postures and prevent a child from taking weight within his own base and keeping his feet plantigrade. Development of walking is prevented as standing and weight shift by the child himself is disrupted by the wheels. The child will therefore sit into the canvas or hang on to the rim of the walker and clutch it with tense bent arms. There are walking aids which suspend a child from an overhead bar in a parachute design between his legs. Weight bearing is taken through both plantigrade feet and as some of the suspension lifts the child's weight off his feet, there is less hypertonus and better weight shift.

Children who run headlong are most likely to hang on the rims of any wheel walker and run dragging their feet. Their walkers should be weighted or a brake applied to the back wheels or, best of all, remove all wheels. Remind these children to walk slower and practise more standing still with feet together or as little apart as they can manage.

Grasping with one hand is usually a progression from walking holding on with two hands. However, if the child takes weight abnormally through one side more than the other or if there are asymmetrical postures, then *two* aids need to be used, until he walks alone. Some children progress to grasping one *clumper* or stick in the centre and in front of them, instead of using two aids.

A child 'walking on his hands' and *'hanging on his armpits'* in walking aids so that he hardly takes weight on his feet should be discouraged from doing so. If not he will step in this way for years and his independent walking will not have any opportunity of developing. Give extra training in all aspects of head trunk and pelvic stability in both standing and sitting development for these children.

Abnormal postures of the head, trunk and legs need to be corrected as much as possible (Figs 7.170–7.179). If correction is not possible with a particular walking aid then a better one should be found, or perhaps walking with aids not trained at all. In such cases rather train the earlier levels in the development of standing or walking more thoroughly.

Note Pushing a trolley with handles which are too low or sticks and clumpers which are too low may increase head and back rounding.

Walking aid giving too much aid Always assess the child's own ability to weight bear, step, control head, trunk and pelvis, and grasp before supporting him in these abilities.

RISING TO STANDING (0–12 months)

Prone to standing (Fig. 7.180) At earlier developmental levels the child has learnt to roll over and get on to his hands and knees or rise from prone on to hands and knees (0–6 months). Train him to rise to half-kneeling then to standing (6–12 months); see Prone development (Fig. 7.184).

Supine to standing Rising from supine to sitting into squatting on both or one foot and pulling up to standing may be easier for the child. Help him to develop this by taking both his hands when he is sitting on the ground. Stabilize his foot with your foot and wait for him to pull himself forward over his feet and then extend his legs. The full rising can be carried out from supine to squatting and up to standing by holding the

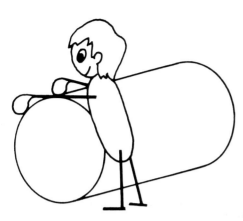

Fig. 7.180 Assume standing from prone lying across a roll, large ball or bed. Check that heels are on the ground, knees hips straight and, if necessary, turned outward.

child's hands and feet flat on the table. Hemiplegic or asymmetrical children can be encouraged to take weight on the more affected side as they squat and rise (see Supine development; see also Fig. 7.184).

Sitting to standing   Rising from sitting on a chair (Fig. 7.181) or from squatting to standing (Fig. 7.182) can be carried out with manual resistance applied on the top of the child's thighs. The child's thighs should be kept apart and in external rotation by the therapist who is either behind or in front of the child. If the therapist sits on the ground in front of the child she has the advantage of making sure that his weight comes forward and well over his feet. Getting the child's *nose over his toes* is important or he will not become independent in rising. He will tend to use an extensor thrust or get up abnormally by pushing on his feet, leaning backwards and grasping your hands, being totally dependent on you in

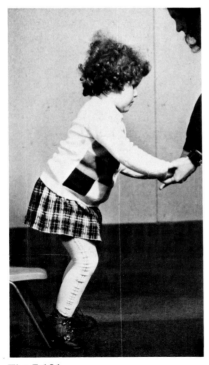

Fig. 7.181

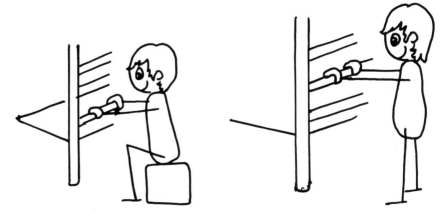

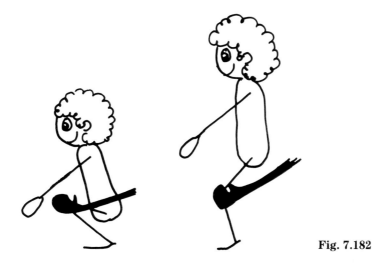

Fig. 7.182

order to rise to his feet. He may learn to bring his own weight forward
over his feet if he is also told to reach forward and down to the floor and
raise his bottom off the chair. In some children resistance may be given
at the lumbar area to augment this movement. Rising from the floor and
from a chair to standing can be taught by careful verbal instruction. For
example, rising from a chair involves: 'Put your feet flat on the ground,
bring your nose over your toes, lift your bottom, stand up'. Rising from
kneeling to standing (Fig. 7.183) holding crutches or other walking
aids to standing. Other rising problems have to be solved in individual children. Figure 7.184 gives various sequences for rising reactions.
Slow rising and hold prepares for attainment of squatting in next
stage.

12–24 Months normal developmental level

COMMON PROBLEMS

Delay in walking alone, improvement in walking pattern, e.g. narrower
base, arms coming down from being held up in abduction, steps more
rhythmical, equal, smoother, standing alone and play in standing, rising to
standing completely on his own, starting and stopping his walking, stair
ascent and descent, use of inclines and walk on rough ground improves
until second and third years.

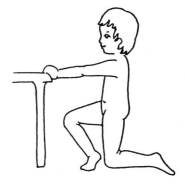

Fig. 7.183

Abnormal performance A variety of Abnormal gait patterns in the
walking child, see the section on abnormal gait above.

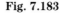

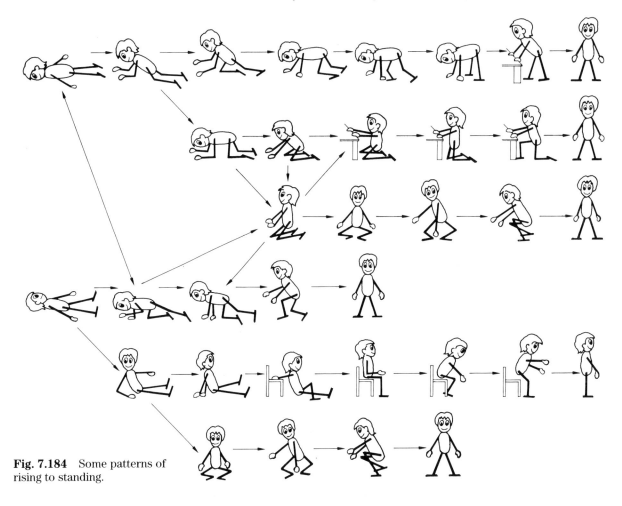

Fig. 7.184 Some patterns of rising to standing.

Reflex reactions The following are expected at this level:

(1) Saving from falling by staggering (protective) reactions in lower limbs, forward, sideways, backward, crossing over and hopping; also upper limbs as before.

(2) In standing, tilt child backward resulting in trunk flex forward and dorsiflexion of feet – forward results in back extension, rise onto toes, laterally results in trunk incurving towards the upright, inversion of one foot, pronation of the other.

(3) Rotate child in standing, feet apart, results in one foot inversion to the rotated side, the other foot in pronation.

(4) Arm saving reactions become more established in all directions.

TREATMENT SUGGESTIONS

Gait   See Figs 7.170–7.174, without support.

Other techniques   See above 9–12 months level but without walking aids.

Stair climbing is also dependent on standing on one leg long enough for the other to deal with the step. This should be trained on and off a low box, progressed to higher boxes as well as staircases, pavements, and ladders.

Train walking and stop, walk and turn, walk between and round objects, walk on different terrains. Walk backwards. Run holding child's hand. Stoop, stand, pick up toy, re-erect; stand, kick and throw balls.

Train staggering reactions   Hold child's arm and push and pull him in all directions to provoke staggering or hopping reactions (Fig. 7.185). One foot may be held instead and the child pushed forward and a protective

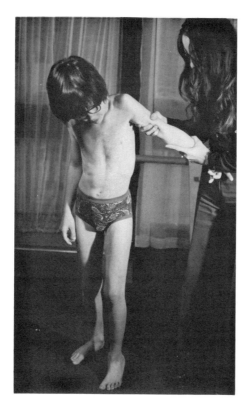

Fig. 7.185

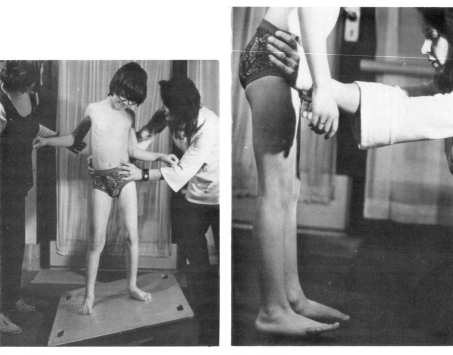

Fig. 7.186   Fig. 7.187

Fig. 7.188   (a) Counterpoising on one foot. (b) Variety of benches for stepping over, walking along and sitting activities.

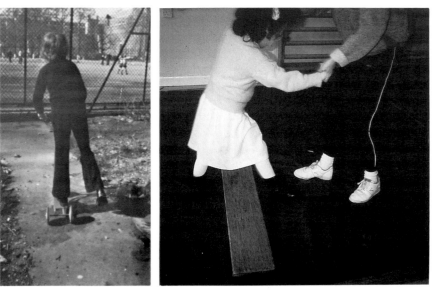

a   b

step provoked. Also hold hips and sharply rotate child to provide a protective step.

Tilt reactions (Fig. 7.186)   Tilt the child back, side or tilt him at his hips (Fig. 7.187):

- To provoke tilt reaction in trunk with large tilt over.
- To provoke reaction in his feet. See also Chapter 9 on the treatment of valgus feet.

Carry all these out against manual resistance – 'Don't let me push you'.

More advanced counterpoising on one foot is shown using a scooter (Fig. 7.188a) and when stepping over benches or toys of different heights (Fig. 7.188b) as well as in activities such as climbing and kicking balls (see Tables 7.1–7.5).

2–7 Year levels (Tables 7.1–7.5)

Train tricycling (Fig. 7.189), hop, skip and jump and the variety of activities at the different developmental levels described in the work of Gesell and others (see Table 7.5).

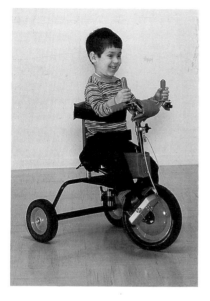

Fig. 7.189   An adapted tricycle for handgrips, trunk support knee extension-flexion and dorsiflexion (acknowledgement to Rifton Tricycle).

Table 7.1   Motor developmental stages, 2–7 years (based on Cratty 1970; Gesell 1971; Sheridan 1975).

2 years
Climbs on to furniture
Pulls wheeled toy by string
Ascends and descends stairs holding on, two feet per stair
Gait pattern changes from wide base, short, flat foot steps to narrower base, more heel–toe action established by 3 years
Arms held in abduction during gait come down to relaxed flexion at child's sides
Legs change from external rotation to facing forward
Walk, run and stop alone
Avoids obstacles while running or walking, steers wheeled toys
Throws ball without good direction and excessive effort
Arms held out when asked to catch a ball
Walk backwards, sideways, between obstacles
Walks into a ball to attempt kick

2·5 years
Jumps two feet together
Ascends stairs, holding on, alternate feet
Descends holding on, two feet per stair, ascends two feet no hold
Steers tricycle while 'walking' his feet on ground
Stands and kicks ball with one foot
Stands on tip-toe by imitation

Table 7.1 *Continued.*

3 years

Ascends stairs, no holding on alternate feet
Descends stairs usually two feet per stair, no holding on
Jumps from bottom stair or pavement
Climbing furniture, apparatus well
Runs and turns, runs and pushes large toys
Walks on tiptoes, on heels, heel–toe action in walk up inclines, uneven ground
Balances on one foot alone, momentarily, enough to walk on line unsteadily
Pedals tricycles and pedal cars
Imitates movements, e.g. wiggles thumb, asymmetrical arm position unless very complicated

4 years

Throws and catches ball with more control, less effort, more direction and does not need to place arms out to catch
Bounces ball, picks up ball or object with bend from waist
Walks on wide balance beam, near ground, walks heel to toe on line steadily
Stands on one foot 3–5 seconds alone
Hops on right or left foot increasing distance
Imitates finger plays including fine pincer actions
Gait pattern now with arm swing, as adult: stops suddenly; turns on the spot

5 years

Climbs trees, ladders, apparatus
Expert at sliding, swings, 'stunts'
Dances, hops and skips to rhythms
Throws and catches ball in various directions, smaller balls
Kicks ball on the run
Counts fingers by pointing

6 years

Wrestles, tumbles
Roller skates
Jumps rope, begins skip with rope
Stands on one foot with eyes closed
Bounces and catches balls

7 years

Walks on narrow and high balance bars
Throws ball about 30 feet
Begins team sports

Movement development shows improvement in speed, precision and decrease of effort or extraneous movements. Increase of endurance. Perception of space, timing and rhythm become integrated with many of the motor skills, see physical education literature for further details and for patterns of performance.

Table 7.2 Character sketch of developmental stages, 1–7 years. (With acknowledgements to Dr P.M. Sonksen from her thesis (1978) for MD entitled: *The neurodevelopmental and paediatric findings associated with significant disabilities of language development*, The Wolfson Centre Library, University of London, Mecklenburgh Square, London WC1.).

Item	Stage by age (years)	Stage 1	Stage by age (years)	Stage 2	Stage by age (years)	Stage 3	Stage by age (years)	Stage 4	Stage by age (years)	Stage 5
Gait in walking	1·6	Early toddler	1·9	Late toddler	2·3	Young child heel strike	6·0	Adult. Heel toe push off		
Upstairs	1	Creeps on hands and feet	1·9	Walks 2 feet/step + hand. Exaggerated foot lift	2·3	Walks 2 feet/step + hand. Economical foot lift	3·0	Walks 1 foot/step and hand	4·0	Walks 1 foot/ step. No hands
Downstairs	1·3	Sitting bumps or creeps backwards	2·0	Walks 2 feet/step + hands (giving much support)	3·0	Walks 2 feet/step + hand	4·0	Walks 1 foot/step and hand	4·6	Walks 1 foot/ step. No hands
Toes	2·0	Balances momentarily but lowers heels to floor before walking	2·6	Walks on toes but with much ↑↓ movement of heels which touch floor often	3·6	Walks well on toes with no ↑↓ movement of heels	4·6	Runs well on toes		
Heels	2·0	Toes raised when standing but lowered to floor before walking	2·6	Walks with toes raised and whole forefoot off floor only for some steps	3·0	Able to walk on heels with forefoot only occasionally sinking	3·6	Walks well on heels		
One foot preferred	2·0	Tries but unable (may *cheat* by holding on to something)	3·0	Momentarily succeeds 0–2 seconds	4·0	3–9 seconds	5·0	10–12 seconds	6·0	12–16 seconds
Hopping preferred	2·0	Unable – may jump up and down 2 feet together	3·6	1–4 hops	4·0	5–8 hops	5·0	9–12 hops	6·0	Over 12 hops

Note   Ages given are in years and months.

Table 7.3 Developmental stages of the catch, 1–8 years (after P.M. Sonksen).

Stage I: boys 1–1·6 years/girls 1–3 years
In this early stage the child may either make no attempt at all to catch the ball, and merely let it hit against his body again and again, or else he may arch his body backwards and extend his arms fully forward meeting in the midline, and with hands wide open. The child looks directly in front of him, but not at the ball or at his hands; he does not follow the ball path nor make any anticipatory movements to catch the ball, and never catches the ball. His only reaction is one of blinking on being hit by the ball.

Stage II: boys 2–5 years/girls 2·6–5 years
The child is looking at the ball and prepares himself for the catch by extending his arms forward, now separated by a few inches, flexing his elbows slightly, hands very slightly cupped, and may arch his body forwards before or during the catch. The child manages to catch about half of the balls which are thrown directly into his arms by trapping it between his chest and his arms.

Stage III: boys 2–6 years/girls 2·6–>7 years
The child now holds his arms forward in a more relaxed fashion than the previous stage; there is more flexion of the elbows, the arms are more widely separated, hands slightly more cupped, and the body arched slightly forward. He watches his hands and follows the terminal part of the ball path into his hands, making some anticipatory movements of his arms to catch the ball. The child now manages to catch all balls which are thrown directly into his hands.

Stage IV: boys 4–>7 years/girls 4·6–>7 years
A more relaxed posture is now assumed; the child watches the thrower and keeps the arms more widely separated from each other, elbows flexed, hands relaxed with fingers now slightly opened out. The knees may be kept slightly flexed. The child moves his eyes appropriately to follow the greater part of the ball flight from the examiner to his hands, and makes anticipatory movements of the arms and body to catch balls which are thrown to the side. He now manages to catch about half of the gentle side-throws by clapping the ball and holding it or by stopping and re-routing it to catch it between his arms and chest.

Stage V: boys 4·6–>7 years/girls 5·6–>7 years
The child is now fully relaxed and with elbows flexed by the side of the body, hands relaxed and fingers open; the eyes and the arms are well coordinated and he follows the ball path throughout, making the appropriate body and arm movements earlier than at Stage IV. All direct and side throws are now being caught by the child.

Table 7.4 Developmental stages of the throw, 1–8 years (after P.M. Sonksen).

Stage I: boys <1–1·6 years/girls <1–3 years
The child at this early stage may adopt one of three ways for effecting a throw. The most common way is by holding the ball with both hands in front of his chest, keeping elbows flexed. He then stoops, straightens and heaves with his whole body and lets go of the ball, expending much energy for little force of throw and poor direction. In the second variety the child effects the throw from the same position as just described but delivers by suddenly extending his elbows in overhand fashion and releasing the ball at the end of elbow extension. In the third variety trunk rotation alone, unassisted by shoulder movement at this stage, brings forward the abducted arm which holds the ball, and the child releases the ball at the end of the swing; in this variety one arm is used. Neither leg is usually brought forward in any of these three forms.

Stage II: boys <1–4·6 years/girls <1–4·6 years
The throw at this stage is effected through a shoulder movement. Neither leg is advanced usually. Sometimes the child starts walking holding on to the ball in one hand. He then suddenly stops walking and at the same time swings his arm/s forward at the shoulder joint, keeping the elbow extended in an underarm or overarm delivery, less commonly sidearm. The accuracy of the throw is still erratic in height and direction, but is delivered with somewhat greater force than a Stage I throw. About half the children will use both their arms and deliver in underarm fashion usually, in an upward or backward direction depending on the point of the arc where the ball is released.

Stage III: boys 1·6–6 years/girls 2–6 years
The main movement at this stage is sudden forward flexion of the elbows, usually underarm assisted by a forward flexion swing of the shoulder. Usually the body is arched forwards slightly, and neither leg is advanced in the majority of the children. A significant proportion, however, advance the ipsilateral leg, which is kept extended at the knee throughout the throw, and receives the body weight towards the very end of the throw. More children use one arm, usually the right, rather than both.

Stage IV: boys 2·6–>7 years/girls 3–>7 years
A flick of the wrist now assists the throwing movement and improves height control. The execution of the underarm throw at this stage is slower than the previous stages. Neither leg is usually brought forward, but again a significant proportion advance the ipsilateral leg, and less commonly the contralateral leg. The vast majority of children deliver in underarm fashion, but when the contralateral leg is advanced an overhand throw at just above shoulder level is effected through an elbow extension and wrist flexion at this stage. The vast majority of the children now throw with one arm, usually the right.

Stage V: boys 3–>7 years/girls 3–>7 years
Individual finger movement and perfect timing of release of the ball at this stage contribute to the performance of a mature throw with good control of height and direction. The fingers do not move as one unit but rather in a rapid succession of flexion movements at the m-p joint starting from the little finger and moving on to the index. The body is arched forward and there is dropping of the throwing shoulder before delivery; during delivery the body weight is shifted forward on to the advanced leg, which increases in flexion at the knee during this weight shift. Proportions vary between the sexes in the choice of leg advancement. Half the boys bring the contralateral leg forward, one fourth the ipsilateral and the other fourth neither. Three-fourths of the girls advance neither leg, and one fourth advance the ipsilateral leg.

Table 7.5 Developmental stages of the kick, 1–8 years (after P.M. Sonksen).

Stage I: boys <1–2·6 years/girls <1–3 years
The child walks, runs, or *straddle-toddles* towards the ball, and then walks into it, displacing the ball rather than actually kicking it. Some children who are standing near the ball or have come to a stop near it, lift up one foot and then step on to the ball. Children at this stage sometimes overbalance and fall.

Stage II: boys 1·6–>7 years/girls 2·6–>7 years
From a standing position the child propels the ball forward by flexing the leg at the hip and maintaining his balance on the other leg. If the child has run to the ball, he will stop just in front of it, adjust himself and/or the ball, and then kick the ball.

Stge III: boys 1·6–>7 years/girls 2·6–>7 years
The child can now run towards the ball and kick it whilst running, propelling it forward with some force and good direction. He anticipates the kicking position and brings the supporting leg at the side of the ball before swinging the kicking leg forward. The latter leg is not kept fully extended throughout the kick, but is kept slightly flexed during the swing and then fully extended for the actual kick.

Stage IV: boys 4–>7 years/girls 5·6–>7 years
The child and the ball are moving towards each other, and the running child can now kick the oncoming ball with good direction and force. He can anticipate the slight modification of the ball's position moving towards him as he brings himself to the kicking stance, and he hits the ball end on, suddenly reversing its trajectory towards the examiner.

DEVELOPMENT OF HAND FUNCTION

The development of hand function not only depends on the motor control of the shoulder girdle, arms and hands but also on visual, perceptual, perceptual-motor and cognitive development (see Table 7.6).

The *main motor aspects* of hand function involve the type of grasp, the pattern of reach, the pattern of reach-and-grasp and the pattern of release (see Table 7.6). These aspects may develop independently of the gross motor activities in prone, supine, sitting, standing and walking development. Although this discrepancy of motor levels appears, it is essential to develop this fine motor ability as:

(1) Use of hands is helpful for perceptual development, cognitive development and for the emotional satisfaction of the child.
(2) Use of hands is particularly important for the handicapped child for support on open hands or grasp so that he can hold on and sit, stand, walk or pull himself into any position.
(3) Hands can be used to help establish shoulder girdle fixation which is fundamental to many of the fine and gross motor skills.

Table 7.6 Development of hand function and eye–hand coordination.

0–3 months
Eye-to-eye contact (parallel eyes)
Fixes eyes on light; eyes follow object to midline (1 month), to past midline (2 months) over 180° (3 months), down, then up eye movement
Hands opening from closed posture
Reflex reactions: Tactile grasp; stretch grasp; blink; doll's eye reflex. Moro, ATNR, reflex hand flare open

3–5 months
Grasps with his eyes when interested in object
Hand regard or studies his hands, brings hands together in midline, clutches and unclutches hands
Visual exploration of environment, visual directed reach begins
Clumsy reaching, bilateral; corraling an object
Clutches clothes, touches body, mouth, face
Grasps object placed in hand; adducted thumb
Reflex reactions: Moro, ATNR disappearing, absence of grasp reflex

5–7 months
Reaching successfully in all directions, depending on trunk balance
Bilateral reach, unilateral reach; excessive MP/finger extension
Grasps feet in supine and sitting – bilateral then unilateral; thumb pressed into opposition
Maintains grasp (grip) on stationary object
Ulnar grasp changing to palmar grasp; wrist flexed becomes straight
Mirror movements of grasp in the other hand
Moves head to see things, eyes converge and focus on pellet at 10 feet; smaller pellets seen by 9 months (Stycar tests); rakes pellet with flexing-adducting thumb
Continues to mouth everything, hand to mouth movement with object
Reflex reactions: Saving and propping downward, forward and beginning laterally; posteriorly later (12 months)

7–9 months
Transfers object from hand to hand
Unilateral reach and grasp; wrist extends
Radial grasp, beginning use of fingertips with opposed thumb
Holds one block while given another
Offers cube, but cannot release it; drops objects
Releases cube by pressing it against a hard surface
Bangs two objects together; compares them
Pats, bangs, strokes, clutches, rakes, scratches – pats mother's face, pats image of face in mirror; thumb abducted or opposed

9–12 months
Protrudes index finger, pokes objects with finger, other fingers flexing
Grasps between fingers and thumb then one finger and thumb (crude to fine pincer grasp)
Pick up and place in and out of large containers; places lids
Reach and grasp possible in all directions, with supination and other improved control of arm; appropriate anticipatory grasp
Release with gross opening of hand then more precise until places small objects in jar, peg in hole, for appropriate anticipatory release
Looks for fallen toy (permanence of objects); casts toys
Reflex reactions: Saving and propping backwards behind child; lateral and oblique

Table 7.6 *Continued.*

12–18 months
Casting of toys stopping; mouthing stopping
Watches small toy moved across room up to 12 feet
Builds tower of two cubes; places pellet into bottle
Pushes and pulls large toys
Drinks alone from cup, often spills

18 months to 2 years
Delicate pincer grasp and release
Takes off shoes, socks, vest, hat
Turns pages of book
Strings large beads, later smaller beads
Scribbles with pencil; whole hand grasp, supinated
Feeds self clumsily
Hand preference more obvious

2 years
Pencil grasp, pronated fingers, wrist deviates
Throws ball inaccurately
Unwraps sweet
Screws and unscrews lids, toys
Imitates vertical line; scribbles and dots

3 years
Takes off all clothes, puts on most clothes
Feeds self completely, using fork
Copies circle; static tripod pencil grasp
Draws a man simply
Cuts with scissors
Washes alone

4 years
Draws simple house, more detailed man
Brushes teeth, dresses alone except for buttons and laces
Constructive building, including three steps with cubes
Matches and names four colours
Copies cross; static tripod grasp modified

5 years
Copies square, triangle, letters; dynamic tripod pencil grasp
Matches 12 colours
Drawing and copying improved
Uses knife and fork
Dresses and undresses completely

Note Assessment measures of detailed hand function interwoven with conceptual, perceptual and ADL development are carried out by occupational therapists and psychologists. (See also the Physical Ability Assessment Chart in the Appendix, and sections on Developmental stages, Feeding, Dressing, Play and perception in Chapter 8.)

It is, however, impossible to concentrate on hand function without considering the many direct relationships of gross motor development to the acquisition of hand function. These important relationships are:

Upper limbs and the postural mechanisms

(1) Establishment of head control is important for hand/eye coordination.
(2) Establishment of postural fixation of the shoulder girdle is obtained when leaning on elbows or on hands in various gross motor activities in prone, supine, sitting, standing and walking development. This helps shoulder fixation for reach, reach-and-grasp, and to coordinate manipulation or activities such as pouring liquids.
(3) Establishment of head, trunk and pelvic postural fixation and counterpoising in sitting and standing makes it possible to use the hands other than in lying or only if the child is firmly tied to a chair. Thus training of all the counterpoising activities in prone, supine, sitting and standing includes training of reach, reach-and-grasp and release (Fig. 7.190).
(4) Development of rising reactions. Hands and arms are used to help in

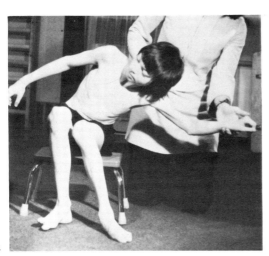

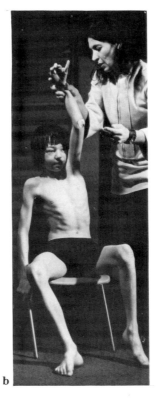

Fig. 7.190   a, Absence of counterpoising in the trunk leads to child falling over the arm during its movement. *Note* attempts to counterpoise with the better arm or by grasp may occur. Encourage this only if trunk counterpoising is totally impossible. b, The trunk is counterpoising the arm movement. Patterns of arm movements should be trained together with counterpoising, in all positions. *Note* the height of the chair controls the position of the legs. A lower chair should be used to prevent any extensor spasticity, to stabilize the child or diminish athetosis.

a   b

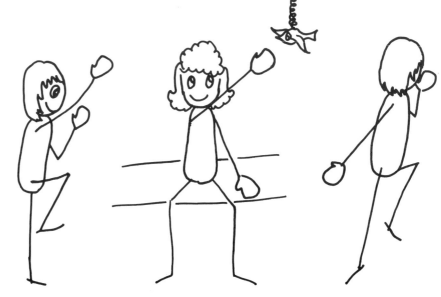

Fig. 7.191 a, Arm pattern of shoulder flexion-adduction-external rotation trained within training of rolling. b, Arm pattern of shoulder flexion-adduction-external rotation as a reaching pattern. c, Arm pattern of shoulder extension-adduction-internal rotation within rolling prone to supine, or within creeping pattern in prone, may be used in reaching back and behind child as, say, in putting on a coat.

the change of various postures or the assumption of posture in gross motor development.

(5)   Development of saving reactions in the arms. The upper limbs are thrown into various patterns involving active contractions of the muscles in synergies (patterns), to save and prop the child as he falls off balance. Although the hands and arms participate in *automatic* saving and propping reactions as well as in various rising reactions, these will not necessarily contribute to *voluntary* movements. Voluntary movements of reach, grasp and release have to be specially trained in fine motor activities.

(6)   Many of the arm synergies trained in gross motor skills are those used in voluntary reach (Fig. 7.191). However, these patterns need to be practised in the context in which they are used.

Upper limbs and abnormal motor behaviour

(1)   Abnormal postures of the whole child include abnormal postures of the arms and hands (Fig 7.192–7.194). Correction of the whole child often corrects the arms. Also corrective arm patterns improve the rest of the child (Fig. 7.195).

(2)   Involuntary movements in the hands or whole arm disrupt hand function. These involuntary movements may stem from the whole body. There may be involuntary motion in another part, say the 'kicking about' of legs only, which disturbs the use of the hands.

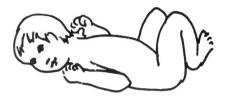

Fig. 7.192 Shoulders protracted or retracted with arms flexed-adducted and hands clenched in a predominantly flexed child similar to the newborn. Inability to reach out or can only reach near his body. There is associated difficulty of release if hands flex or clench excessively.

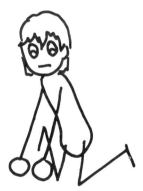

Fig. 7.193 Arms flexed-adducted and internally rotated with elbows flexed and pronated, wrists flexed or mid-position and hands clenched or open. Shoulder flexion-adduction-internal rotation may also occur with elbow extension-pronation. Shoulder flexion-adduction may also occur with elbow supination and flexion in athetoids who *fold their arms in* towards their bodies in supination, with hands open or clenched.

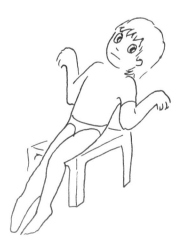

Fig. 7.194 Arms held up in the air in abduction-external rotation, elbow flexion and supination with palms facing toward the child. Elbows may also be flexed and pronated with palms facing outward. Hand may be hanging down or clenched; this is also called the *bird-wing position* and is seen in supine, sitting and standing positions. This may alternate with an asymmetrical tonic neck reaction or other asymmetry. There is inability to reach forward, bring hands together and develop *hand regard* and bring hands down for support.

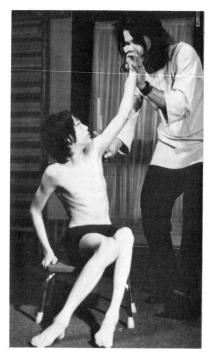

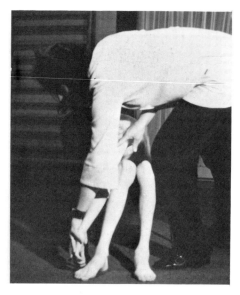

Fig. 7.197 Arm elevation-abduction-external rotation corrects abnormal patterns in Figs 7.192–7.194 and is used to reach out for an object, to dress or brush hair (elbow flexion/extension).

Fig. 7.198 Arm pattern adduction-internal rotation corrects abnormal arm pattern in Fig. 7.194 and is used to reach down for an object, dress, wash and other functions.

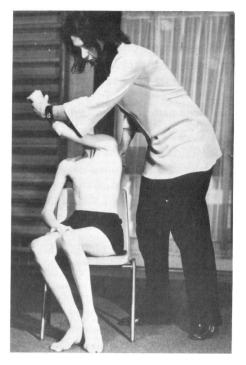

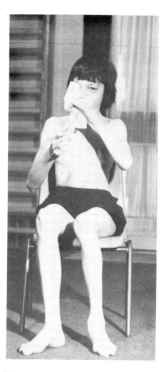

Fig. 7.199 Arm pattern flexion-adduction-external rotation corrects arm patterns in Figs 7.192–7.194 and is used to reach for an object, touch own face, blow nose, dress or eat.

Fig. 7.200 Arm pattern in use for wiping nose or face.

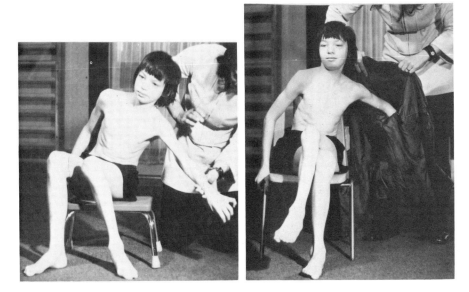

Fig. 7.201 Arm extension abduction-internal rotation corrects arm patterns in Figs 7.192–7.194 and can be used for dressing, reaching out and pulling trolleys in play.

Fig. 7.202 Arm pattern in Fig. 7.201 in use for putting on a jacket.

Reach and grasp are also carried out in these positions. Trunk rotation with reaching must be included, especially if resistance is given to the child's arm movement.

Direction of reach is first low down in front of child, forward at shoulder level, to the side, above him, and then behind him. This progression is easiest for most children.

Facilitation   These patterns can be facilitated with:

(1)   Touch, pressure stretch and resistance and good rotation of the child's shoulder girdle and/or trunk.
(2)   The therapist may manually rotate the shoulder girdle, pull shoulders forward or backward to initiate automatic arm pattern (see Figs 7.63 and 7.64 as examples; see also section on Creeping patterns in prone development, 0–3 months stage).
(3)   The child can be taught to reach to food, for toys or take part in a play activity selected to provoke the use of specific arm patterns (Fig. 7.196).
(4)   The child can be asked to concentrate on the arm pattern, e.g. 'stretch your arm up and back', 'stretch your elbow'.

(5)   The daily activities of feeding, dressing, washing, bathing may use many desirable arm patterns including those described below, if activities are carefully trained.

Vision and arm patterns   It is important to stimulate the child's visual development and to associate it with development of hand functions, e.g. encourage child to look at hands or object he is reaching for during facilitation of arm patterns.

Unilateral and bilateral arm patterns must be included in the programme. For example:

(1)   Unilateral patterns such as moving one side only; leaning on one

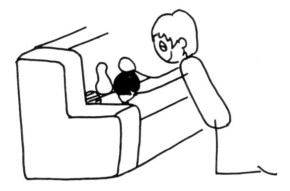

Fig. 7.203   Both arms stretch towards toys and palms face inwards to hold toys. In this way elbow extension, supination is correcting the abnormal postures. *Note* the rest of the body is also correcting abnormal postures associated with abnormal arm postures. Use of *both* arms corrects asymmetrical ability in arm function as in hemiplegia.

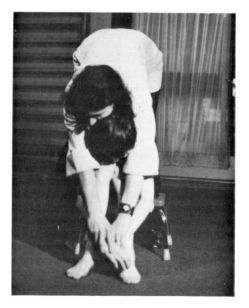

Fig. 7.204   Bilateral arm patterns against appropriate manual resistance in diagonal patterns. Note facilitation of wrist extension.

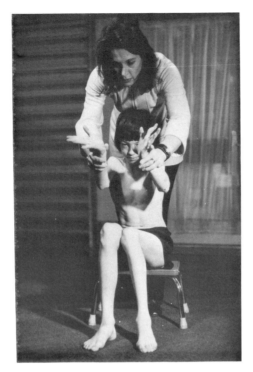

Fig. 7.205 Bilateral arm patterns against appropriate manual resistance in diagonal patterns. Note facilitation of wrist extension.

hand and move with the other; grasp a support with one hand and move the other (asymmetrical work) (Figs 7.197–7.202).

(2) Bilateral patterns with the child's arms in the same direction (bilateral and symmetrical) for support and for motion. This takes place to counteract abnormal asymmetry of posture of arms and body, and of function (Figs 7.203–7.205, see also Fig. 7.195). Use of less affected arm together with affected arm may help the latter.

(3) Bilateral patterns with arm, in opposite directions (bilateral and reciprocal). This takes place in creeping, reciprocal arm swing, or motion using play equipment, pulleys or hand pedals.

(4) Bilateral patterns with each arm in a different direction, e.g. one sideways the other forward (bilateral and asymmetrical) which is used in advanced perceptual motor training and for highly complicated counterpoising activities and hand skills.

ABNORMAL HAND GRASPS AND
TREATMENT SUGGESTIONS

(1) Abnormal grasp may be present in association with the total abnormal posture or only with the arm posture when the rest of the body functions well.

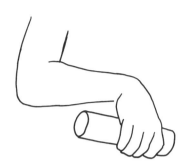

Fig. 7.206 Common abnormal pattern of arm, wrist and hand.

(2)   Grasp may appear to be abnormal because it belongs to a lower level of development.

(3)   Anticipatory grasp is distorted by inability to open clenched hands and by intellectual delay.

Treatment suggestions for some abnormal grasps

Grasp only possible in one position of the child's arm   Train grasp within all the corrective arm patterns (above, in different directions, and body positions).

Wrist flexion with palmer or pincer grasp or inability to grasp in this position (Fig. 7.206)   Press the child's wrist down as he tries to grasp; place the object above the level of his wrist; ask him to lift his hands to the object, see Figs 7.205 and 7.208. Some children may need a wrist splint to train grasp with wrist in midline or extension (dorsiflexion). In some spastic children, the wrist extension should only be to the midposition as there is excessively tight finger flexion with full wrist

Fig. 7.207   Abnormal grasp with excessive finger flexion and no flexion or even with hyperextension of metacarpal-phalangeal joint is being corrected by the therapist in **b** during grasp and release.

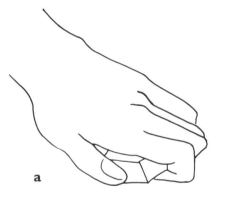

a

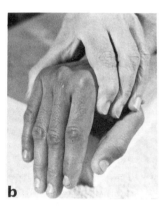

b

Fig. 7.208   Overcoming excessive wrist flexion, overflexion of fingers by the task selected and the therapist pressing the wrist down. Press on a child's wrist as he grasps bars of walkers, spoons, cups and other tools.

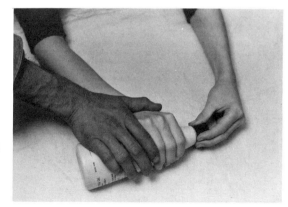

extension. This also prevents the child from opening his hands to release the object held. The use of glove puppets, hammering, lifting dowels out of holes, rings off a stick and similar activities may help to obtain wrist extension for grasp and release. In some cases, grasping with the wrist in extension may be achieved at the cost of opening the hand in this particular position. The child may then discover he can open his hand if he palmer flexes. It is preferable to train hand opening correctly, see below, 0–3 months level, and later release, 9–12 months level.

Excessive finger flexion in grasp   With or without hyperextension of the metacarpophalangeal (m-p) joints (Figs 7.207 and 7.208). Place the child's hand over thick, larger objects such as bars and handles. Do not use squeezy toys. Hold the dorsum of the child's hand, lift his mp joints and he or you can then press his fingers straight over the large ball, box or square bar. This may de done with the child's mp joints pressing on the edge of a table as he tries to hold on to the edge, or the solid edge of a truck or windowsill. Counteracting this abnormal grasp will prepare him for grasp with his fingers straight, using finger tips later. Grasping edges of cards or lids is one way of training this straight finger grasp.

Adducted thumbs and ulnar grasp   The adducted thumb may grasp or be useless. It can be seen with ulnar grasp (Fig. 7.206). In some children the ulnar grasp may result when the child tries to compensate for or avoid the adducted thumb. When the thumb is abducted a radial grasp may occur. In other cases, the child grasps his fingers in midposition with an adducted thumb. Adducted thumbs may also accompany palmar flexion, or excessive finger flexion with hyperextended mp joints. The child should be encouraged to move his hand towards the thumb side, for example he pushes rolling toys away towards the radial side; brings a spoonful of food towards his mouth and other activities which encourage him to move his hand towards the thumb side. He may not manage this unless you hold his hand in midline during grasp. Hold the child's hand between his thumb and forefinger on one side and hold down the ulnar side as he grasps (Fig. 7.209).

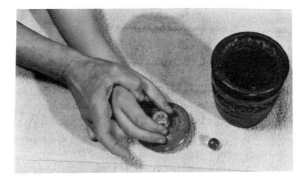

Fig. 7.209   Guided abduction of thumb and pincer grasp.

The little finger and ring finger may be bandaged if the child does not resent such a procedure. Training grasping of objects with the radial side is then encouraged. Check that the child is not given handgrips on walkers, handles and other supports which encourage an abnormal ulnar grasp. The handles at the sides of rollators or on crutches may do this. Avoid the angled spoons for handicapped children as they create an ulnar grasp. The child's adducted thumb may be abducted-extended if he tries the above suggestions. Also use techniques for hand opening (Figs 7.195–7.197, 7.201 and 7.205).

Adducted thumbs may be held out with thumb splints made from pigskin or other splints (see Appendix). To get an adducted thumb out of a fist or hand, never pull it by its tip or you may dislocate or sublux the mp joint. Sometimes the other fingers flex more as you do pull on the thumb. Rather turn the whole arm or forearm to face palm up to the ceiling and abduct the thumb out from its base. It is important to follow this procedure with placing the child's hand over a toy teaching him a palmar grasp or later a radial grasp. See Opening of hand techniques.

Anticipatory grasp The methods to reduce tight fingers and thumb contribute to opening of the hand to anticipate the size of object for grasping. More experiential learning is still needed.

Inability to grasp with both hands simultaneously Although this is normal in many children under the 6 months developmental level, it may also be due to:

(1) Lack of head control in midline so the child uses the hand that he can see; lack of midline head control is seen in persistent head turning to one side, which occasionally improves spontaneously.
(2) Asymmetrical tonic neck response to one side which is 'used' to reach and grasp to that side.
(3) Hemiplegia or greater spasticity or weakness of one arm in any diagnostic type.
(4) Excessive spasms or involuntary motion on one side, rare hemiathetoids.
(5) Sensory loss on one side especially astereognosis in the hand or visual field defect, usually in some hemiplegias.

Inability to grasp on one side will often be associated with *inability to use both hands together* or to hold with one hand and carry out an action with the other. During training of prone, supine, sitting and standing development check that both hands are given objects to grasp simultaneously or to grip for support. Use play activities which require two hands, e.g. play in water and washing, sand, clay, dough, larger toys, handles on bowls, rolling pins, sieves, sticks with dangling bells, broom, bicycle pump, toy concertina, small cymbals, maracas or toys which make a noise if pushed at both ends (Fig. 7.210).

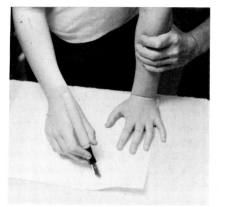

Fig. 7.210 Support on more affected hand pressed open whilst child uses more skilful hand. Affected hand stabilizes the paper or toy during use with the other hand.

Associated grasping or clenching on the affected side when grasping with the unaffected or the less affected side. This is usually seen in spastic children; associated *mirror* movements of the hand not in use are normally seen in very young children but disappear on normal development. If these mechanisms persist they can prevent the child's transfer of objects from hand to hand and holding with one hand while using the other hand. Hold the more affected elbow straight with hand flat on the table while the other hand grasps. Have the child lean on the more affected hand held open, with the weight on the elbow or hand. Carry out joint compression to facilitate support on this hand as the other hand is used actively. Practise activities which include each hand in a different action, e.g. hold toy with one hand, carry out action with the other, winding a bandage or hold support with one hand, and use a variety of movements with the other.

Other parts of the body may also tense or assume abnormal postures during grasp. Check that these associated reactions are corrected as well. Correct positioning of the rest of the body during hand function will control this.

PRACTICAL POINTS IN TRAINING GRASP

(1) Use of the eyes must be associated with development of hand function. Follow the developmental levels below.

(2) Normally the grasp reflex and hand clenching disappear before voluntary grasp develops. Do not wait or work on total disappearance before putting the object in the child's hand to grasp. Use techniques (below) to open the hand just before methods to develop palmar grasp, in the same session.

(3) Children should not grasp in association with any of the abnormal arm postures shown in Figs 7.192–7.194, e.g. grasp with wrist and/or elbow flexed, shoulder adducted and flexed. Use the arm patterns suggested in Basic arm and hand patterns for all levels of development. Check that the rest of his body does not assume abnormal postures as he grasps.

(4) Have the child hold objects with his hand in pronation, then later in midposition and still later in supination. However, some athetoid children may start with grasp in supination and then midposition and finally in pronation.

(5) Make sure that the child looks at the object in his hand. Talk about the object at his comprehension level. Encourage his speech during the use of his hands if this does not distract him.

(6) Check that he is interested in the object placed in his hand. Always have him choose from an array of objects which help his function.

ABNORMAL RELEASE AND TREATMENT SUGGESTIONS

Total inability to let go of an object placed or grasped by the child after 5 months.

Release only possible if wrist is flexed The child may use his other hand, his chin or even his forehead, or a hard surface to press the back of his hand to obtain this flexion (palmar flexion).

Release against a hard surface after 11 months of age. These problems of release are discussed in the appropriate developmental levels below.

Release with thumb adducted and flexed in palm Train a release with thumb abduction with a supinated forearm. Sometimes external rotation from the shoulder is indicated. Thumb splints may help. Movements to train hand opening also contribute to keeping the thumb out of the palm. Supination of the child's forearm by the therapist facilitates thumb extension or abduction.

Release with ulnar deviation can be improved if objects are released into container or dowel holes on the radial side of the hand.

Release with excessive splaying of the fingers, i.e. hyperabduction with hyperextended metacarpalphalangeal joint. A similar pattern is also seen in normal babies casting objects at about 11–15 months of age. In addition this pattern is seen in avoiding reactions in the hands of athetoid children. There may also be plantar and/or a visual avoiding reaction with the avoiding reaction in the hands caused by tactile and visual stimuli respectively. Grasp smaller objects and train release into a defined area or container. Hold the ulnar side of the child's hand and train release on the radial side and later with thumb and finger. Training more precise release is closely allied with the training of pincer grasp below (Fig. 7.209).

Hand and visual avoiding reactions can be helped if one introduces the object for grasp and release slowly into the child's visual field and into his hands. Encourage him to maintain his grasp to make him less sensitive to the stimuli.

Conflict between grasp and release This problem is seen in an athetoid child when he makes attempts to grasp an object but immediately withdraws his hand, splaying it open. This presents itself as a repeated involuntary motion in the hands. This conflict between the grasp reflex and the avoiding reactions was described by Twitchell (1961). To break this disabling conflict, it is advisable to reinforce the child's active grasp or grip. Encourage maintained grasp for as much of the day as possible on bars, handles, in front, at his side, above or below him in his various situations during the day. When he is sitting on a pot he should grasp a bar, sitting in a pram, he should grasp a bar, standing and using walkers or hold sticks vertically or frequently carry around a rod grasped in both or one hand.

Other involuntary motion disrupting reach and grasp Train conscious control of reach, grasp and manipulation. With practice the involuntary motion is mastered by a child to a greater or lesser degree. Help the child by having him use his hands while leaning on his forearms, or reach to toys through a thin padded hoop which limits the excursion of the involuntary motion. Wide uprights of, say, a play pen also limit his involuntary motion as he reaches between them for toys.

Note It is important to carry out all the training of reach, grasp and release as suggested below under the appropriate developmental levels. The patterns of reach, grasp and release may only be retarded in some children. This means the pattern may be a normal one but seen at an earlier age than the child's chronological age as in children with severe learning problems.

All the patterns of grasp and release are also disrupted by visual loss, any sensory loss in the hands, as say in hemiplegia, and by lack of visual, perceptual or perceptual-motor development as seen in intelligent 'clumsy' children.

Stages of hand function development

0–3 Months normal developmental level

COMMON PROBLEMS

Delay in eye focusing, visual fixation, visual following of an object. Clenched hands not opening; thumb still held in palm.

Abnormal performance, see abnormal patterns of arms and hand above.

Reflex reactions Grasp reflex, Moro reaction, tonic neck reaction, sudden flexor or extensor spasms.

TREATMENT SUGGESTIONS AND DAILY CARE

Eye focus and following (hearing and vision)

(1)   First offer visual interest in the midline and help the child keep his head in midline. You may need to hold both his shoulders forward, occasionally backward to allow him to keep his head

upright (see sitting development, vertical head control; prone development, head control).

(2) At first place your face or toys close to the child's eyes, about 8 inches (20 cm) from him.

(3) Eye-to-eye contact is of first importance before interest in objects. This should be done at the child's eye level whether he is in side-lying, supine, prone, supported sitting or supported standing.

(4) Associate vision, hearing and head control with face-to-face singing, talking. Vary tones of voice. Encourage baby's smile and general communication.

(5) Help him to look at and follow shiny, moving, colourful noise-making mobiles, toys, fishes in a tank, marble runs, a torch light, switching the room light on and off. Use coloured ribbons, Christmas decorations, shiny bottle lids or other bottle tops strung together, rattles.

(6) Use red, yellow or primary colours, not pastels.

(7) Use jingling noises and not high pitched or sudden loud noises as the child may still have a startle reflex.

(8) Hang tinkling bells, jingling beads or mobiles in the window or doorway so that they move and make a sound as the wind blows. Encourage his early crude arm reaching movements at 5 months level or even earlier stages (von Hofsten 1992).

(9) Encourage the child to look and see where the noise came from, to listen to your voice. Put him in different positions, i.e. prop the child up in sitting as well as lying on his back, side or stomach to carry out the above.

Also see Opening of hand, treatment suggestions below and in other motor developmental training, for example:

(1) Hand may open within the arm pattern of elevation-abduction-external rotation, or extension-adduction-internal rotation in techniques of creeping, and then, if possible, used in prone development, in supine, side-lying, sitting or standing (Figs 7.191, 7.195–7.197, 7.201 and 7.205).

(2) Weight bearing on elbows and/or on hands decreases hand clenching, see prone, sitting, standing development which include leaning on elbows or hands.

(3) See correction of postures in all developmental levels – as these also correct arms and hands.

3–5 Months normal developmental level

COMMON PROBLEMS

Delay in hand regard, visual exploration; bringing hands together and to mouth, touching self, unable to grasp object placed in hand, grasp and shake toy, no clumsy reaching for objects. Grasp is normally on ulnar side at this level. The clutching of child's hands on clothes on himself or mother may be delayed. Hands fully opened.

Abnormal performance

(1) Asymmetrical bringing of hands to midline, reach or grasp.
(2) Touching with semiflexed or closed hand.
(3) Abnormal patterns in reaching (see abnormal patterns, arms and hands above).
(4) Abnormal grasp (see above) except ulnar or lateral grasp, at this stage.

TREATMENT SUGGESTIONS AND DAILY CARE

Hand regard and bringing hands to midline Positions to bring arms forward are:

(1) Place the child in side-lying or lying in a hammock, or half-lying in a sack of polystyrene beads, with shoulders brought forward or in supported sitting with arms held forward. Whenever possible have child sitting and leaning with his body against the table or your lap, his arms placed well forward. These positions offer more opportunity than supine for bringing his arms to midline level with his eyes. Only in those cases when the child *can* bring his arms forward is it advisable to have him in supine. A side-lying board is helpful for those children who persist in keeping their arms in abnormal positions at their sides, out of their view (see Supine development, Fig. 7.70).
(2) Once his hands are in front of him the child can be made aware of them by your talk, shining a torch on them, putting sticky things such as jam on his hands, playing with his fingers, putting thimbles, rings, coloured ribbon, bracelets or bells on his wrist and fingers. Help him open his hands and rub his palms together, touch his face and body and later clasp and unclasp hands, clutch materials and toys which are soft and easy to clutch.

Expect him to combine reach and grasp alone. See 6–9 months level in prone development, for taking weight on hands: used also in sitting and standing development. See also stimulation of saving reactions in prone, sitting and standing development.

7–9 Months normal developmental level

COMMON PROBLEMS

Delay in transfer from hand to hand, unilateral reach and grasp, grasp more than one block at a time, radial grasp, hand patting, banging, clutch, stroke, rake, scratch, bang two blocks together, release against a hard surface, use of hands in feeding and in holding on during sitting and standing. *Scissors* grasp (inferior pincer grasp) and use of fingertips. Delay in anticipatory grasp in relation to size, shape, weight of object (9 months) (von Hofsten & Ronnqvist 1988).

Reflex reactions

(1) Saving and propping reactions expected.
(2) Abnormal persistence of reactions from previous levels.

TREATMENT SUGGESTIONS AND DAILY CARE

(1) See above for reach and grasp patterns.
(2) Train own grasp in feeding, dressing, washing, toileting (Chapter 8). Begin training release by having the child release a block against a hard surface with the heel of his hand held down against the surface, or his other hand or his body. Release may be impossible if hand opening has not yet been developed. See methods at 0–5 months level or training of hand opening.
(3) Ulnar grasp now develops into radial grasp.
(4) Transfer from hand to hand, banging blocks together and also holding on with one hand or leaning on one hand during unilateral reaching are particularly important for hemiplegic children, and any child with asymmetrical postures.
(5) Play with suitable toys, dough, sand, water can involve transfer from hand to hand, grasping more than one object at a time as well as patting, banging, clutching, stroking, raking, scratching and release against a hard surface.
(6) Patting with open hands may become a persistent pattern in some children with severe learning problems. Activities involving grasp and manipulation at the child's developmental level counteract these and other *mannerisms*.

9–12 Months normal developmental level

Delay in finger/thumb opposition and development of crude and fine pincer grasp, no protrusion of index finger. Release of objects, casting haphazardly and delay of increasing control into containers, building two-cube tower, look for fallen toy (permanence of objects). Supination may not develop. Delay in developing anticipatory grasp.

Abnormal performance See abnormal arm posture, abnormal reach and grasp (above). Abnormal arm patterns prevent increasing control of shoulder, elbow and hand. Abnormal grasp prevents pincer grasp, and index finger approach.

Reflex reactions

(1) Excessive avoiding reaction may prevent release becoming controlled as well as preventing grasp (casting toys is normal at this level of development).
(2) Saving and propping backwards is expected at this level.

See training of reach and grasp, especially grasp in supination.

Index finger approach to objects isolated finger pointing and pressing.

(1) Help the child to use toy telephones or ordinary telephones, using his index finger for dialling.
(2) Use index finger to press into dough, plasticine or sand. Later make lines and scribbles in sand.
(3) Put paint on finger tip and make dots and scribbles.
(4) Press-studs on clothes should be attempted. Press small button or knob which obtains interesting sound or visual appearance as, say, a jack-in-the-box or other pop-up toys. Help him switch electric lights on.
(5) Use finger puppets.
(6) Play the keys of a piano, typewriter, cash register or with an abacus.

Pincer grasp Begin with larger objects then progress to smaller objects. Thumbs and all finger tips are used first before thumb and one finger, usually the index is used. (Crude and fine pincer grasp.)

(1) Pick up small sweets and place in container or in his mouth. The child may like to pick up buttons, wooden beads, marbles, under

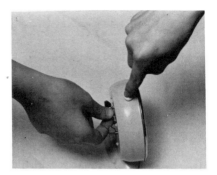

Fig. 7.211 Developing index finger pointing and pressing and a fine pincer grasp during action of pull, push and later to turn object, as in screwing movement.

supervision as he may pop them into his mouth to swallow them.

(2) Hold thick crayons and if possible pencils and thick chalk for making marks on paper or later writing (Fig. 7.210).

(3) Use toys with small knobs and of small size for fitting shapes.

(4) Hold small cup handles for drinking.

(5) Wind clock and turn its knobs, press alarm bell to stop, press doorbells. Various toys have knobs and buttons to press and turn.

(6) Begin screwing action with large screw-toys, lids, etc. (Figs. 7.208, 7.211); progress to medium and fine screwing later.

Allow the child to attempt the activities on his own. If he cannot manage to isolate his index finger, hold his little, ring and middle finger flexed for him until he can do this alone (Fig. 7.209). Use *finger plays* for index finger and touch finger to thumb games. Make spectacles, blow soap bubbles, say 'how do you do' and *walk* fingers. Develop a greater variety of grasps (Fig. 7.212).

Continue training release This involves dropping objects (beanbags) into container on the ground below his chair, in front of his chair, at the side and behind his chair. Help him look and see 'where it dropped'. Later encourage him to place small objects in smaller containers until he learns to fit a peg in a formboard, and build one block on top of the other. Precise release is required for building a tower of blocks as well as perceptual and conceptual adequacy. Building blocks may be made of sponge rubber shapes, wood, plastic or be household objects, boxes, tins or pots, to develop the child at this level.

Manipulation and perception/conception Manipulation is by now integrated with perceptual development of:

(1) Space and depth in, say, well coordinated reach and grasp activities.

Fig. 7.212 Some hand grasps: to take hold of and to grip. Spherical with palm or fingertips only, hook grasp, cylindrical grasp. Others are lumbrical (Fig. 7.208), pincer (Figs 7.209, 7.210) with sides and with tips of fingers. *Remember* to train grasps in vertical, pronated, supinated and other hand positions.

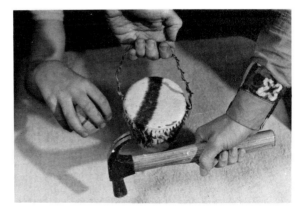

(2) Form in placing a round peg in a round hole and similar matching.

(3) Size in placing small objects into large containers, arrange according to size, etc.

(4) Colour and shape in use of matching toys (but not naming them), such as various posting boxes, mosaics and other sorting activities, jigsaws.

(5) Discrimination of soft, hard, scratchy, smooth sensations.

(6) Other conceptions in social activities; wave bye-bye, point to visual stimulus, pat own face in mirror and smile at himself, and play pat-a-cake.

Perception, conception and fine motor manipulation continue to develop in such activities as threading large beads, smaller beads, other threading toys, scribbling, drawing, painting, pasting, using pegboards, draughts, jigsaws with knobs, sorting buttons, shells, using sewing cards, and a large variety of constructional toys, screwing toys, posting boxes and many more suggested in toy catalogues and by the Toy Libraries Association. Eye–hand coordination and rhythm, speed and precision of movement will need to be developed further after the basic arm and hand actions are trained (Morgenstern *et al.* 1966; Cratty 1967, 1969; Brereton 1971) (see Appendix).

Chapter 8
Motor Function and the Child's Daily Life

Chapter 7 has presented ways in which the child may develop various postures, maintain these postures during movement, or disturbance of balance, get in and out of postures, obtain various forms of locomotion, and acquire the use of his hands. All these motor functions are used in the child's daily life and a few are summarized to demonstrate their use in self-care, perception, speech and language and socialization. The child's mental and emotional development are also involved as they interact with a child's achievement of motor abilities. It is also important to consider many recreational activities which can also be condusive to improved motor and sensory function, e.g. swimming, horse-riding, skiing and so on (see Leach 1993).

Motor function and feeding, dressing, toileting, washing, bathing, play and communication

Those below are of particular significance although all motor functions are needed (see Levitt, 1994).

Vertical head control in midline and slightly forward.
   Obtained by: holding the child's shoulders forward with your arm when he sits on your lap when a baby; or next to you on his chair when older. Facing the child and holding his arms stretched forward across the table between you or holding him in weight bearing on his forearms. With his grasp and trunk leaning against the table or forearm support the child may do this alone.
   This is especially needed for being fed, feeding himself, communication, visual exploration and other functions.

Sitting on the floor and/or sitting on a chair of the correct size and design
   Obtained by: sitting, leaning trunk against table, box or pouffe or other support, leaning on forearms and feeding, drinking, washing his face, playing, pulling off a jumper and so on (Fig. 8.1). Support is also possible by having the child grasp a rail or horizontal bar attached to the table, the wall, the bath, the toy shelves during daily activities (Fig. 8.2). Sitting astride his own chair and grasping its rungs may also be useful for communication, play, dressing and feeding. The child's one arm may be

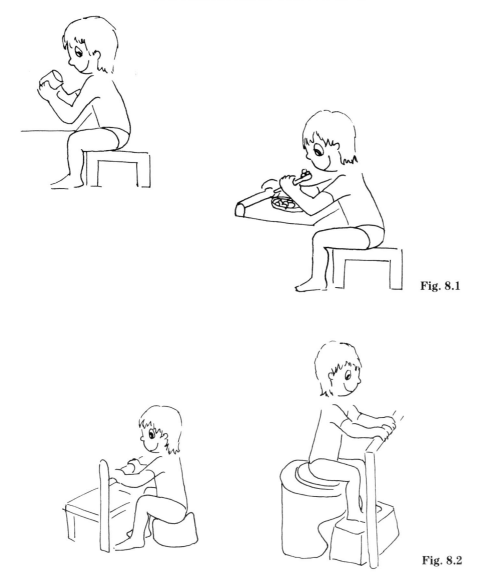

Fig. 8.1

Fig. 8.2

released for any activity, whilst his other controls his balance. Support may be needed for some children from behind by an adult sitting there and holding the child forward with her own body or her hand or by stabilizing the child's pelvis with her knees, or with her feet and knees if she is sitting at a higher level to the child.

Sitting with support to the child's pelvis may be carried out with groin straps, diagonal strap across the hips or by firm pressure with your hand in the lower area of the child's back, or holding his hips. The child can then carry out any particular activity using head, trunk and hand control.

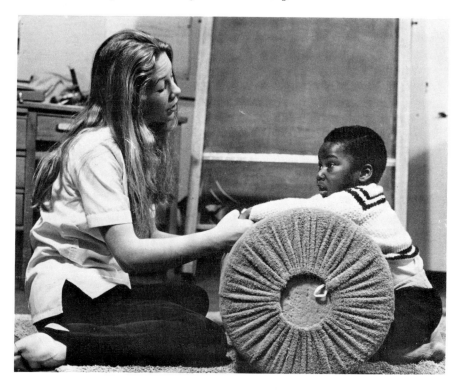

Fig. 8.3 Speech therapy associated with control of excessive extensor thrusts of head, trunk and legs, asymmetry by correct position. Vertical head control and face-to-face communication is promoted. Grasp is developed.

Sitting against a wall, in a room corner or on a variety of chairs may be used for particular children. Do not let the child slump or slide down during activities.

Correction of abnormal postures is needed so that the child can function (Fig. 8.3).

Prone and head control is used for play, communication, or when being washed, dressed or having a nappy changed in babyhood. Some use this for chewing, sucking and swallowing to increase action of the muscles against gravity.

Obtained by: use of wedges, rolls, over your arms or lap, prone standers.

Standing or kneeling upright, holding on to tables, rails for painting, drawing, washing, toilet for boys, dressing, communication and many other play activities.

Obtained by: use of horizontal, sometimes vertical, rails on tables, walls, blackboards, easels, leaning against stable furniture, holding rungs of a chair or use of various standing frames, prone boards attached to tables.

On hands and knees may be needed for play with cars and trains, gardening, housekeeping activities, sandpits, painting.

Obtained by: cushions, wedge cut out to fit a child, over adult's lap when sitting on the floor, or have the child on a crawler which is stabilized. This position is *not* advisable for those children who sit back on their heels during the activity or who have tightly bent hips and knees.

Use of the hands is obviously required for all activities and cannot be condensed unless a particular activity is discussed in detail.

Motor function and perception (Cratty 1969, 1970; Ayres 1979; Penso 1987)

All the training for motor function is also training perception. Thus during the motor developmental techniques the therapist should recognize and involve the following main features:

Tactile recognition and discrimination of textures, temperatures. Also feeling different shapes, sizes, weights, to develop stereognosis. Meanings of words are also associated with these experiences of say smooth, hard, scratchy, knobbly, rough, hot and cold. Later matching and discriminating of these sensations develops.

Recognition of the child's own body by tactile recognition during motor training as when touching his mouth, face, grasping his foot or clasping his hands, as well as touching others and sitting close to others.

During motor training, communication and other activities the child can learn his body parts by having his nails painted, putting on rings, bells, bracelets, make-up moustaches, earrings, ribbons, bandages, thimbles or lighting up parts of his body with a torch. When handling the child in movement training rub, stroke, or use ice as well as words to draw attention to parts of his body. Use of vibrators is also valuable.

Drawing attention to the child's body parts leads to an awareness of his own spatial relationships or body scheme, i.e. where are his toes? – in front, below, and so on. This is also involved with his body planes (Cratty 1969, 1970) and which part of his body is moving and in which direction. Although this is experienced through sensation and proprioception, it need not be made conscious during motor training unless this conscious awareness is helpful to train movement itself or to train perception. This verbal, visual and proprioceptive linking is considered of importance by psychologists, teachers and physical educators, for the child's future educational activities.

Intersensory development is encouraged by associating the movements trained with hearing and vision. During the training of hand function there is obviously linking between what the child grasps, feels, sees and even tastes and smells. Manipulation of objects with banging, throwing, squeezing, rolling, mouthing, breaking are linking many senses. This leads to another related perceptual experience, which is:

Appreciation of the qualities of objects and of their relations to one another With gross motor activity and fine motor activity the child should be helped to recognize round, square, long, cylindrical shapes and discover which fits into which, which can be placed on top of which object and also which object is nearer, further away, or behind, in front of or next to the other. These perceptions and concepts are part of education and occupational therapy and must be presented to children through various activities. Motor training overlaps into these areas.

Appreciation of the child's relationship to objects and space These perceptual experiences also become involved with motor function. As the child learns to move through space he is also learning to appreciate how far he is from objects, how to get into and out of things, how to get on top of, under, around, behind and many other relationships to objects and space.

Thus the child finds out about his body parts, their relations to each other and also the relations of his body to objects and to space during gross motor development and fine motor development.

Development of praxia, motor planning or using the movements appropriate to a motor task such as dressing, writing, using a pair of scissors or other implements. Although this depends on perceptual experiences and on the training of the neuromuscular system and is helped in its development during motor developmental training, it could be defective on its own in brain damaged children.

Specialized perceptual and praxic training (including visuomotor training). This may still be needed for many specific problems found amongst motor handicapped children. These problems occur despite general perceptual experiences included in the motor developmental training. The specialized therapy and education needed is discussed elsewhere and advice must be sought from psychologists, teachers in special education and occupational therapists (Morgenstern *et al.* 1966; Ayres 1979; Presland 1982; Fisher *et al.* 1991; Steel 1993).

Although special sessions of perceptual-motor training are needed it must be remembered that *perception is also being trained within the activities of feeding, dressing, washing, bathing, toileting and especially playing*, and is part of the programme.

Motor function and speech and language

All the motor developmental training should be associated with words related to body parts, movements and the purpose of motor functions. Colours, shapes, sizes and all the other perceptual and conceptual experiences integrated with motor functions are greatly involved in development of speech and language.

Motor functions have already been summarized above for positions for communication, for feeding, for play, as well as other daily activities. All this promotes speech and language as well. The development of feeding develops the use of the oral musculature needed for speech. In addition, breathing exercises and stimulation of the facial muscles with neuromuscular techniques of touch, pressure, stretch, and resistance may be helpful. Short periods of ice application, or ice lollies reduce spasticity of tongues or mouths and promote speech. Quick ice stimulation of the mouth muscles may help 'flabby mouths' and make the child aware of his muscles of speech. This discourages dribbling by provoking mouth closure so facilitating swallowing. A large red handkerchief pinned to the child's clothes has motivated some children to remember to wipe their mouths and remember to swallow and keep lips closed. Unobtrusive pressure across the area between nose and upper lip or sometimes just below the lower lip provokes mouth closure and makes swallowing possible, instead of dribbling. Drooling is normal until about 15 months of age.

The development of speech and language requires special advice and treatment from speech therapists (Levitt & Miller 1973; Latham 1984; Stroh & Robinson 1991).

DEVELOPMENT OF COMMUNICATION — BRIEF SUMMARY

(Hearing, speech, language and communication.)

0–3 months   Use of cry, facial expression. Stills to noise. Smiles at mother.

3–4 months   Sounds vary and beginning to babble.

4–6 months   Babbling, begins some intonations. Watches adult's lips. Turns to sounds; to mother's voice. Laughs, squeals, chuckles, annoyed screams. Excited limb motion as social responses.

6–8 months   Lip and tongue sounds. Syllables (baba a ba) begin.

8–12 months   Double syllables, first word. Turns to sounds that interest him instantaneously. Vocalizes to make personal contact. Associates sound with movement. Playful turn-taking.

12 months   Understands more than expresses. Follows adult's simple direction ('Give me', 'No'). Responds to his name. Single word. Real object labels.

12–20 months   Imitates adult speech. Echolalia. Two- or three-word phrases. Responds and discriminates sounds, speech, simple commands.

24 months Loves listening to stories, jingles; verbal explosion.

3 years Simple sentences, many questions. Give own name. Nursery rhymes, talks to himself. Normal stutter. Unique dialogues.

PRACTICAL SUGGESTIONS

(1) Follow general guide of developmental levels and individual assessment by speech therapist and psychologist.

(2) Always try to communicate with the child with noises (at first not too loud and sudden), songs, smiles, gestures; talk near the child and with face-to-face contact.

(3) Speak slowly and distinctly but not with exaggerated articulation, as in 'baby talk'. Wait for any response by the child.

(4) Say names of familiar objects, colours, what they are used for, and demonstrate and name parts of the body, and talk of child's own experiences.

(5) Child should be able to see your face in a good light during speech. Try to be at his eye level whenever possible.

(6) Play lip and tongue games, lick off jam, lollies, peanut butter and during feeding use babbling and speech and stimulate child to do so.

(7) Encourage child to participate in songs, rhythms, body movements and hand finger plays. However, do not pressurize the child to speak but create informal situations for conversation, especially in groups.

(8) Use gestures, facial expressions, but not if speech is possible. Make it rewarding for him to use speech or have a need for speech by having to ask for things, indicate things, and so on.

(9) Praise but do not fuss about the child's attempts to speak and give him time to express himself. Do not finish sentences for him if he can do so in his own time. Do not answer for him if he can say something.

(10) Explore alternative forms of communication (symbolic), e.g. Bliss, Makaton, Paget-Gorman with experts.

DEVELOPMENT OF FEEDING – BRIEF SUMMARY

0–4 months Rooting reaction, sucking-and-swallowing reflex. Hypersensitive mouth or cardinal points reflexes, tongue thrust, open mouth and dribbling.

4–6 months Sucking dissociates from swallowing as child transfers liquids for swallowing. All reflexes disappeared. Bite reflex weak. Takes liquids from spoon. Recognizes bottle.

6–9 months Takes strained foods, solids, bites a biscuit. Holds a biscuit, may crumble in his hand. Up and down jaw motion in chewing, swallows with mouth closed.

9–12 months Finger feeds, chewing with lateral jaw motion, holds and drinks from bottle, from cup with help. Helps mother with spoon to mouth.

9–12 months   Holds spoon alone but cannot bring to mouth with food.

12–15 months   Uses spoon but turns it upside down before reaching mouth or within mouth. Holds and drinks from cup, often spills.

15–18 months   Chewing established. Forward and rotary jaw motion. Feeds self clumsily.

2 years   Uses spoon correctly, occasional spilling, holds glass and cup for drinking, plays with food. Understands what is edible and inedible. Begins straw drinking but bites edge.

2–3 years   Feeds self completely with spoon, with fork. Pours liquids, obtains own drink from tap.

3–4 years   Serves self at table, spreads butter, cuts food.

PRACTICAL SUGGESTIONS (Fig. 8.4)

Unhurried feeding period, to try and give time for the child to actively participate. The speed of your feeding him should be slower and similar to the speed at which his own early attempts will start. Feeding himself and being fed should take place in as social and pleasant an atmosphere of an unhurried meal as you can make it. Speech and babbling in reply to your talk often occurs during such feeding periods. Sitting at meals with the family and other children at school also motivates feeding alone by imitation. Speech may then also occur for the social reasons as well as the fact that eating and drinking activates the speech muscles.

   If the child cannot imitate due to impairments of intellect or vision, or because the others are eating too fast for him to feed himself at the same mealtime, it is essential to have private feeding therapy sessions. There is no distraction and he can concentrate on active achievements. Naturally he should join the others for the mealtimes, but be given something easy to do in the way of self feeding or drinking.

Positioning for feeding should involve an upright position supported or if possible unsupported by special chairs or by the parent. Some feed more easily in a standing frame. See feeding positions in the section on motor function and feeding at the beginning of this chapter. The child's head should be held by you or preferably himself forward and upright whilst taking food, during eating and especially on swallowing. If he is allowed to swallow with his head back over the years, his growing oesophagus will trap food in its longer length and so prove dangerous. Swallowing with head upright also provokes active participation in his training. Gently press his chest to help the head come forward and up and if his head drops give minimal support under his chin. Elbows on the table are recommended! Stability for head and hand to mouth action is promoted and babies and young children with visual disability are made

Fig. 8.4   a, Head extension and tongue thrust interfering with drinking and eating. b, Holding the child's head upright and forward, supporting her chin and stroking under her jaw trains drinking. c, Wait for the child to remove food from the spoon held below her mouth. Keep her head and shoulders well forward as she takes the food.

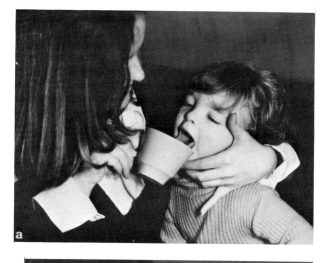

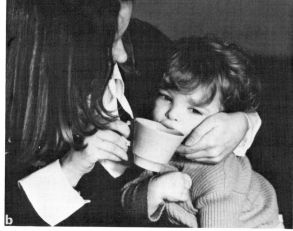

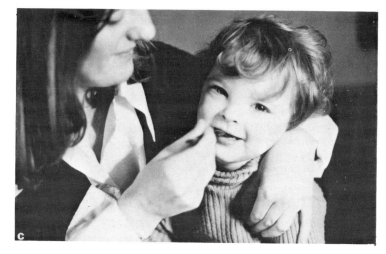

aware of where they find the food and obtain security from the stable table.

Mouth actions in taking the food, keeping the mouth closed during eating, chewing actions and swallowing can be facilitated by your hands, supporting under his chin. Stroke under the chin and along his neck to provoke a swallow whilst your other finger presses his lips closed. Fingers may have to be held above and below his lips to stimulate mouth closure. Simply achieving mouth closure may lead to his own swallow as the food or drink cannot spill out of his mouth. Stimulate chewing by massaging or manipulating the child's cheeks after he takes the small piece of food. Let him take the food off the spoon offered below and in front of his mouth and do not scrape the food and spoon off the top of his teeth.

Weaning from liquids to tolerate various textures, tastes through semisolids to solids is most important and may take longer in some children with disabilities. The visually impaired, the severely intellectually impaired child, and the child with a behaviour problem may be conservative about any change or may use it as a means of controlling the overprotective adults around him. Change from liquids to semi solids gradually by adding to his cup of favourite drink, yogurts, custards, apple sauce, stewed fruit, mashed banana, puddings, crushed fruit in dilution. Gradually transfer to a bowl. Spoon from cup of thickened liquid to spoon from bowl of food as a weaning process. Mashed semisolids enjoyed by a child may have to be mixed with foods he does not like in semisolids and solids. A meal of ice-cream and peas with mince and custard has been known to wean a difficult child to solids! Weaning to solids is not done only to socialize and improve nutrition but chewing solids exercises the articulators for speech. Introduce a solid he can hold and likes in part of every meal from the beginning of training of feeding. Hold an apple slice, a sausage, rusk or cheese. You hold a sliver of meat and teach him to bite whilst you pull on the end of the meat. Always introduce lumps in food by a general 'lumpiness' rather than odd lumps in a smooth sauce, in the initial stages.

Gagging or choking   Keep calm and quickly tip the child forward and down. Avoid banging him on the back. An excessive gag reflex may be neurological and train its control by 'walking' the spoon gradually back on his tongue, give small amount and go slowly giving him time to take the food and swallow. The child may of course gag on foods he dislikes, to which he is allergic or if he has a behaviour problem. He may be reacting against a new person feeding him, an unfamiliar place, especially when in hospital, or he may be seeking the fuss and attention he gets from mother and others if he gags and vomits. Casualness in people's reactions and ignoring his 'performance' may stop this

Fig. 8.5 The child is held flexed for dressing and play. Tailor-sitting is being obtained. Press beneath the big toe and bend hip and knee outward in order to overcome excessive leg extension-adduction for, say, a nappy change, sock removal and getting her into tailor-sitting.

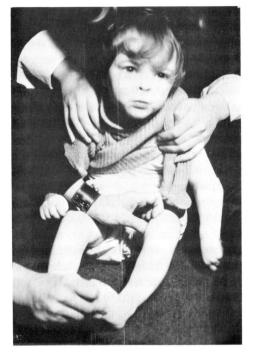

DEVELOPMENT OF PLAY — BRIEF OUTLINE

This is the development of *learning through play*. This is closely correlated with the development of hand function and the development of intersensory relationships and perceptual-motor control.

0–6 months Visual fixation and pursuit, hand–eye coordination and bring hands to midline and grasp, drop, reach and grasp, touch, etc. Play with parts of body, mother's face, nearby materials. Amuses self for short intervals.

6–12 months Rolling, crawling, supported cruising and other gross motor activities to explore, strengthen body generally and enjoy moving. Hand function development using toys or objects. Investigates and experiments with increasing energy.

12 months–2 years Solitary play but imitates another child or adult. Uses large equipment, swings, balls, toys on wheels to push and pull. Sand and water play. Enjoys small objects such as shells, pebbles, buttons – often taken to mouth until 15 months of age.

2–3 years Rough and tumble play. As above only with more perceptual and conceptual ideas. Begins imaginative play ('Let's pretend'). Solitary and parallel play.

3–4 years Plays with other children. Imaginative play, dressing up. As above but not as energetic.

6 years Games with rules, arts and crafts. 'Tricks'.

PRACTICAL SUGGESTIONS

(1) Play differs at different ages, but it is impossible to have it strictly classified as the child's personality, opportunities and intelligence affect this. Social and cultural backgrounds also affect play.

(2) Play is usually a synonym for exploration and experimentation and is a serious affair for the child. Play can also be relaxing, working out emotions, imitating reality in order to understand it in imaginative play, and obtaining satisfaction and development of the child's personality. It is often messy, dirty, untidy and destructive as well as creative and constructive, in the adult sense.

(3) Show the child how to use a toy, but wherever possible see if he can find things out for himself.

(4) Do not interfere with any child who is concentrating on a play activity unless absolutely essential.

TECHNIQUES FOR CARRYING THE CHILD CORRECTLY (Figs 8.6–8.11)

(1) To stimulate head control.
(2) To correct any abnormal postures.

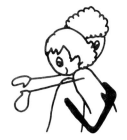

Fig. 8.6 Both the arms are over the adult's shoulder for symmetry, straighten back and raise head. Keep the legs apart, and hips flat if necessary in spastic child. Bring tight arms away from their habitual positions next to the child.

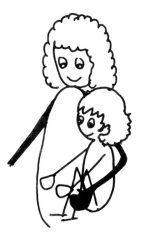

Fig. 8.7 For head control and correcting an excessively extended child, help bring hands down and together helps control an athetoid or floppy child.

lead to deformity. However, not all hypertonic children resort to use of abnormal reflexes to move. Examples:

Opisthotonus or repeated extensor thrusts in the legs only, tends to lead to a fixed extensor posture.

Asymmetrical tonic neck reactions or any other asymmetrical limb postures created by head turning may lead to deformities in the limbs, a scoliosis and/or a torticollis. Extensor postures are associated with asymmetrical tonic neck reactions.

Symmetrical tonic neck reflexes may occur in severe cases. Immobility and lack of treatment may lead to deformities within these patterns.

Reflex stepping may aggravate hypertonic plantarflexors, adductors and extensors if this reflex is used to 'walk' the child frequently.

Excessive supporting reaction may be overstimulated by, say, *baby bouncers* and increases the deformities of the legs, especially equinus and extensor-adductor postures.

Excessive suspension or lift reaction. If the child is lifted or suspended under the armpits and lowered to the ground, and there is an excessive plantarflexion, Tardieu (1973a) suggests this may cause equinus.

Active use of total flexion reactions, withdrawal reflexes in kicking, during rolling, crawling, kneeling. The withdrawal reaction which combines hip-knee and ankle flexion rather than hip-flexion-knee *extension* and ankle flexion may be used in (heel strike) stepping. This hip and knee flexion instead of hip extension-knee flexion or other such synergia may be used in swing-through or push-off in gait. The repeated use of flexion in all these movements or postures tends to flexion deformity.

Use of total extension reflexes as in using the extensor thrust in active kicking, when bounced on the feet in standing, during rolling and creeping along the floor, may lead to deformities into these patterns of extension.

ASYMMETRY

(1) Asymmetrical distribution of hypertonus.
(2) Asymmetrical development of postural reactions.
(3) Asymmetrical presence or persistence of abnormal reflex.
(4) Asymmetrical growth of legs. See abnormal postures and asymmetry in Development of standing, Development of sitting and Prone development.

(5) Hemianopia (of visual field), absent visual acuity or deafness in one ear augments asymmetry.

Any repeated flexor spasms or involuntary athetoid kicking with hip and/or knee flexion, or pawing an athetoid leg may give rise to tightness in knees or hips and knee joints. Similarly and less commonly extensor spasms or rotary involuntary movement may create tightness. Dystonic athetosis is particularly worrying as a cause of deformity.

GROWTH FACTORS

There are four main factors which cause or aggravate the development of deformity.

(1) The difference in leg length, see asymmetry in abnormal postures in standing. (Difference in arm length is not related to the genesis of deformation).
(2) Spurts of growth in cerebral palsied children and adolescents are linked with deterioration and increase of deformities. The unequal growth of bone and muscle, increase in height and especially increase in weight seem to bring on deformities. Usually there would also be less mobility as older children need to spend longer hours at their studies.
(3) The mechanism of growth and spasticity have been studied by Sharrard and by Tardieu & Tabary. Sharrard believes it is the stronger spastic muscles imbalanced with their weaker antagonists, which pull unevenly on growing bones and create deformity. Tabary *et al.* (1972) showed that shortened muscles have a diminution of sarcomeres compared with normally mobile and extensible muscles. The immobile, inelastic, shortened spastic muscles grow abnormally in relation to bone and deformities increase with growth (Tardieu *et al.* 1982). Orthopaedic surgery is inevitable in their view (Sharrard 1971; Tardieu 1973; Bleck 1987).
(4) The specific bony structure of the hip in spastic children does not change as it normally would with growth, due to spasticity and non-weight bearing.

The neck of the femur remains in anteversion and the shaft/neck angle of valgus does not decrease. This is part of the reason for hip deformity, and dislocations.

BIOMECHANICS

Every joint should be considered in the treatment of deformities, whether with or without orthopaedic surgery. This is due to the biomechanics of deformity. The biomechanics which create deformities are not only dependent on the spastic muscle groups, each of which may flex one joint and extend another, e.g. hamstrings, rectus, gastrocnemius, and their relationship to weakness or on the effect on other joints or in the biomechanics of spasticity. The more important clue is the presence or absence of the postural mechanisms of postural fixation, counterpoising and the locomotive reflexes which initiate the step and lateral sway. When these are abnormal the child compensates by using abnormal postures in order to maintain balance in functions such as sitting, standing, crawling and walking. See Development of sitting and standing. Occasionally hip flexion deformity or equinus deformity may disbalance the child, but it is usually the disbalance *of the child* which increases hip flexion in compensation for falling backward (see the Abnormal postures in standing section in Chapter 7).

Therapy and daily care

Treatment aims based on the causes of deformity discussed are therefore:

(1) Motivation of movement throughout the day. However, movements must be varied and where possible of normal pattern.
(2) Frequent changes of the child's posture.
(3) Correct positioning of each part of a child's body in postures.
(4) Postures and movements must include:
  (a) Passive elongation of hypertonic muscles and soft tissues.
  (b) Active and full range of movement of antagonists to hypertonic muscles.
  (c) Active and full range of movement of hypertonic muscles including active work in their elongated position.
(5) Correct any asymmetries of posture, movement or balance and check postural alignments regularly.
(6) Train the normal postural mechanisms and locomotor reactions.
(7) Control recurring involuntary motion in one pattern.
(8) Counteract any relevant pathological reflexes.
(9) Treat the biomechanics of deformity and not just deformity in one joint. As in the discussion of the causes, many of the aims interact with each other.

TECHNIQUES

Techniques for all the aims mentioned above are presented in the sections in Chapter 7 on Physiotherapy suggestions and Treatment suggestions and daily care throughout all developmental stages. There are, however, additional methods which may be required for individual children. These will be offered *with a summary of some of those already mentioned* in the book. It may be helpful to discuss each joint separately, in case one joint is threatening to deform or is already showing more deformity than the others within the total patterns of function. The orthopaedic surgeon usually studies the child for the major deforming factor. In summarizing the methods it may be helpful to remember the following points in connection with the aims of therapy.

Elongation of hypertonic muscles takes place in positioning the child in equipment, in splints, corrective moulds and braces, in plaster of Paris, in orthopaedic surgery. Elongation is made possible by any techniques which reduce hypertonus. Active work of the antagonists to the shortened muscles will also involve elongation of these shortened muscles.

Active and full range of antagonists takes place if the child activates his muscles to hold any of the *positioning* rather than only depend on therapist's hands, equipment, bracing or plasters to hold lengthened position of hypertonic muscles or shortened muscles.

Some workers suggest that there is a reciprocal relaxation of shortened muscles when there is activation of their antagonists. Movements which correct abnormal postures are movements which activate antagonists to the shortened or spastic muscles. They are strengthened and their 'disuse' weakness treated in such movements (Egel 1948; Rood 1956).

Active and full range of hypertonic muscles in movements as well as the above also help to mobilize joints and prevent or counteract deformity.

Reduce hypertonicity In order to obtain the aims of therapy above, especially in relation to the elongation of hypertonic muscles and make it easier to activate their antagonists, it is important to reduce the hypertonicity. A reduction or inhibition of hypertonicity also helps to obtain more efficient muscle action in the hypertonic muscle groups themselves. Reduction of hypertonicity includes the following techniques:

(1) Use of rotation in movements.
(2) Use of gentle *prolonged* stretch in passive movements, equipment, plasters or splintage.
(3) Activation of antagonists on their own or with other methods, may inhibit the spastic agonists.
(4) Ice treatments.
(5) Medical treatments using drugs (McKinlay *et al.* 1980), localized procaine blocks, alcohol (phenol) injections. Total neurectomies are rarely used to cut off nerve supply to spastic muscles, as this also cuts off their ability to work as well. Partial obturator neurectomies may work better.

(6) Vibration techniques (Rood 1962; Hagbarth & Eklund 1969; Eckersley 1990, 1993).

(7) Repeated contractions of spastic muscles to obtain autoinhibition (Rood 1962). An active contraction of the antagonists must follow immediately.

Summary

For a review of orthopaedic surgical procedures see Sharrard (1971), Samilson (1975) and Bleck (1987).

The hip deformities

HIP FLEXION-ADDUCTION-INTERNAL ROTATION

One component may be greater than the others. The shape of the hip joint may be abnormal, e.g. the acetabulum is shallow, neck of femur anteverted; subdislocation and dislocation may occur.

THERAPY AND DAILY CARE

Positioning   Prone lying, legs apart on conical-shaped pommel, in prone wedges, prone board; standing boards, standing frames, standing tables, sitting with legs apart, externally rotated, side-sitting, tailor-sitting, sitting in chairs with pommels; stand or sit straddling equipment of rolls; carrying with legs apart and turned out over adult's hip or over adult shoulder pressing child's hip flat with legs apart.

Splintage and bracing   Abduction pants used in all positions; abduction splint (Fig. 7.115) used in standing and walking; long leg braces with pelvic band; rotation coil attached to pelvic band and shoe for external rotation (but check for any abnormal effect of tibial torsion), *twisters* (Fig. 7.172) for milder spastics (Grenier 1973a).

Plaster of Paris   Long leg spicas to incorporate hip extension-abduction rarely work. Excessive flexor spasms usually occur after removal of plaster.

Ice treatment to reduce hypertonicity.

(1) Apply towels wrung out in chopped ice and water to adductor surface of leg for 3–4 minutes. In addition place the child in tailor-sitting or over a roll *while* the ice pack is tied on to his thighs.

Repeat applications of ice packs. Carry out active abduction movements as well.

(2) Wring rough towels out in ice so that ice flakes cling to the towelling. Roll the whole leg from groin to feet in the towel for 3–4 minutes. Carry out leg patterns with rotation in the hip during and after ice application as well as positioning. Repeat.

Active exercise to antagonists

(1) See developmental training for active hip extension, hip abduction, hip external rotation in creeping, rolling from prone to supine, active extension in 'standing tall', in stand and reach overhead. Counterpoising techniques using leg extension, abduction, external rotation (Figs 7.38, 7.39, 7.168) in four point kneeling and in standing, squatting or sitting rise to standing, kneeling rise to standing, four foot kneeling rise to upright standing, and other postural changes.

(2) Other examples are given in Figs 9.1–9.10. Emphasize the movement of the antagonists to the deformity, e.g. the extensors in flexion deformities.

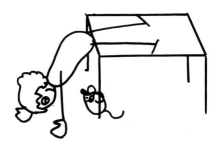

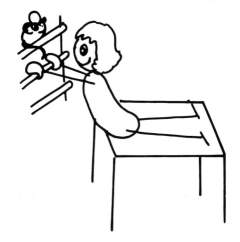

Fig. 9.1 Bend over edge of mother's lap, large ball or couch, raise up and bend down again. Hold rungs and 'walk up' for level hip extension. Keep legs apart and turned out if necessary. Child raises head and trunk up in association with hip extension. Initial support may be given by your hand on his chest. Avoid abnormal extensor thrust.

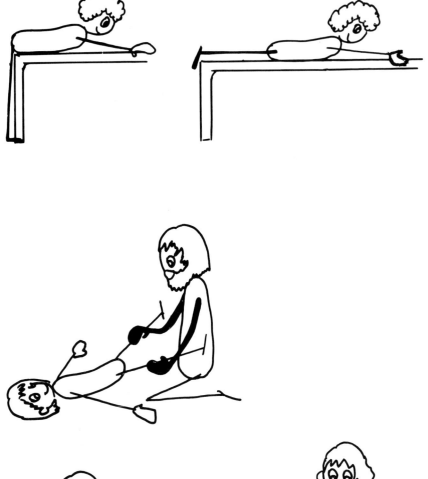

Fig. 9.2 Child's legs over mother's lap, edge of bed, large ball, or roll. Bring legs down to floor (hip flexion) into bed (hip extension). Hold knees and thighs apart in external rotation to encourage hip extension-abduction-external rotation if required. Raise *one* leg at a time to control lordosis (Fig. 9.6). Child may grasp side of table or both his arms are held elevated-abducted and externally rotated by adult if abnormal flexion in arm and trunk is present. Use these movements when getting up on to bed/plinth *or* getting out of bed.

Fig. 9.3 Legs of child held in abduction-external rotation. Active raise of child's hips into extension. *Avoid* use of lordosis to do this. Legs may be on lap of therapist, on low stool or with his feet flat on the ground for 'bridging' the pelvis into extension. Manual resistance may be given to anterior superior iliac spines to augment extension. Obtain flexion by asking child to bend knees to chest then repeat above extension activity. Use this action during play, dressing and washing.

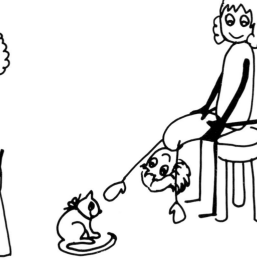

Fig. 9.4 The child actively stretches down and comes up to sitting with or without grasping your hands. For babies you may use the large ball, or roll. The child may also bend sideways to the floor for scoliosis (to side of the convexity). (From Neumann Neurodde 1967.)

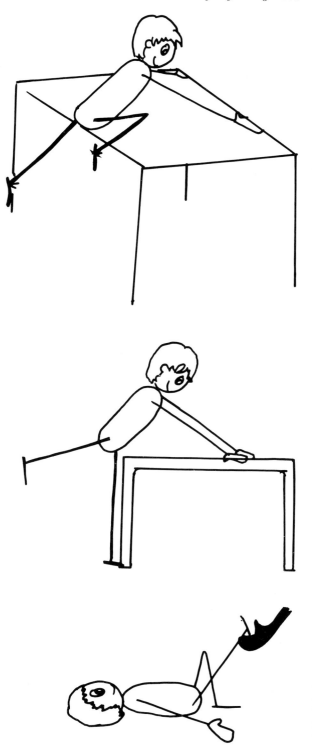

Fig. 9.5 One knee held bent to chest during hip extension of the other leg, to counteract lordosis. Carry this out in side-lying or in prone. Also flex-abduct-externally rotate extended leg for action of those agonists.

Fig. 9.7 One knee flexed to chest or flexed with foot flat. Press other leg into extension into adult's hand, sponge rubber surface, soft couch. Child's hips raise into extension with his weight on one foot. Full flexion of each hip should be carried out actively if required. Arms straight, and hands pressed flat or grasping edge of bed.

Fig. 9.6 Child leans forward onto ball, table, roll, during active hip extension of each leg. Lordosis is more easily controlled this way. Next, flex the leg so that foot reaches high bar or even table.

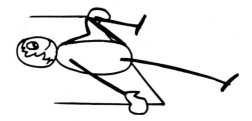

Fig. 9.8 *Activate agonists and antagonists* and full range of active hip and knee motion. Use of arm extension is incorporated in these exercises.

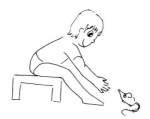

Fig. 9.9 *Activate agonists and antagonists* and full range of active hip and knee motion. Use of arm extension is incorporated in these exercises.

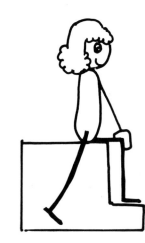
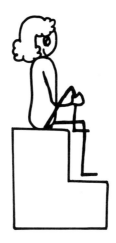

Fig. 9.10 *Activate agonists and antagonists* and full range of active hip and knee motion. Use of arm extension is incorporated in these exercises. Use these movements during dressing/ washing.

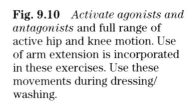

Active exercise to agonists and antagonists   See Developmental training of creeping (flexion and extension of legs), counterpoising techniques in crawling positions and standing position. Sitting, touch floor and raise up in standing, see Figs 9.1–9.10.

Orthopaedic surgery for hip deformities may be: iliopsoas elongation, adductor tenotomies, obturator neurectomies, rotation osteotomies; for hip dislocation: adductor tenotomy and obturator neurectomies or rotation osteotomy or removal of head of femur. Surgeons recommend early weight bearing and abduction *with* extension to prevent subdislocation of the hips in cerebral palsy.

HIP EXTENSION DEFORMITY

THERAPY AND DAILY CARE

Positioning   Chairs to increase flexion, and overcoming extension in standing and walking training, and correct carrying in flexion positions (Fig. 8.7). Use heel-sitting, squatting and crook-sitting.

Splintage and bracing, plasters, ice not used as positioning seems to be simplest and more effective.

Active movements of flexion and of flexion and extension, see developmental training of creeping, crawling and standing (see Fig. 7.173 on correcting hip extension in walking). See Figs 9.1–9.10.

Note   To overcome excessive extension of head, trunk and hips and knees manually and in equipment, it is important to flex the child at his head and shoulders *and* at his hip joint. Hold his head and shoulders, hold under his knees and flex him 'into a ball'. His extensor spasm, thrust or constant extensor hypertonus decreases in this position. This may be easier in side-lying. Try different positions for flexion. *Orthopaedic surgery is not used.*

Knee deformities

KNEE FLEXION

THERAPY AND DAILY CARE

Positioning   Prone-lying with straight knees, sitting with straight knees on the floor, in floor seat or sit on a low chair if back rounds in sitting. Use knee gaiters in sitting and in standing.

A number of research studies including those of Cusick & Sussman (1982) show positive results from the use of below-knee casts. There is progress in foot position, postural alignment, balance and walking pattern.

Application of plaster. Based on work by H. de Rijke, Trengweath Centre, Plymouth, UK, Burns (1970) and Jones (1993). There are many casting materials available and those easily applied and removed, damp-proof and light are selected.

Position Child lies prone with his knee bent so that dorsiflexion is easier to obtain, and to hold as the plaster is being applied.

Personnel One person talks to the child and relaxes him and reads to him. One person applies the plaster and another person holds the foot in the corrected position. To quicken the time taken to apply the plaster an additional helper to cut and soak the plasters is needed.

Preparation of the foot and leg
(1) Clean skin, apply olive oil.
(2) Treat callouses, ingrown toenails and do not apply plaster if any skin abrasions have not yet healed.

Application of the plaster itself
(1) Apply stockinette, then thin cotton wool or orthopaedic bandage, allowing stockinette to hang over toes until plaster of Paris is completed.
(2) Apply compressed felt, with sides trimmed down, to ankle, heel and front of ankle. A shape may be cut so that a piece of felt covers the sole of the foot and the felt then wraps around from the heel to the front of the ankle. Do not overlap felt as this will act as a pressure area or the padding may shift under the plaster if it is too loose. Apply all materials evenly. The orthopaedic bandage may be over felt if this can be more even than under the felt.
(3) Wind wet plaster around ankle first. Do not use a figure 8. The *holder* keeps the foot at right angles or more whilst this plaster hardens slightly. It should be applied with firm tension to hold the foot from slipping.
(4) Apply a plaster from toes to below the knee holding the foot at right angles or more. *Test* that the angle of dorsiflexion used in the plastering can be obtained passively with the child's knee straight. Gradually increase stretch into dorsiflexion in a series for very tight ankles.
(5) Slabs of plaster are put on along the back of the leg up to the toes. The holder keeps the toes *dorsiflexed* and spread out and presses

Use a series of plasters for children who do not maintain correction. Have a short period of exercises and weight bearing before the next plaster is applied. The period between plasters has been from 2 years to a few weeks in different cases. Athetoids should only wear a plaster for a week at a time in case of involuntary movements within the plaster.

Foot and knee plasters have been applied simultaneously by Burns, others prefer below-knee plasters and knee plasters to be separated. After removal of plasters from hip and knee the child often needs exercises, particularly in water, bandaging of knees and treatment of knee swelling as well as long leg caliper.

Cooperation of the parents is essential for good results thus:

(1) Explain the purpose of the plaster and the importance of their help and encouragement to the child to wear the plaster for short periods.
(2) They should check the circulation often, be warned about possible restlessness and have a sedative for the child.
(3) Parents should protect the plaster and allow drying for 3 days. Child may sit with his leg or legs on cushions protected by waterproof material. An old sock, plaster boot or plastic covering may be used to cover plaster.
(4) Parents carry out home exercises and later as much standing and walking as possible.
(5) Discuss with parents which times are convenient for the periods of casting.
(6) Tell parents when the plaster comes off and they should know when their child is coming home with a plaster beforehand, or they may think he has broken a leg!
(7) If child's toes go blue, or if there is extreme pain and upset, the plaster *must* be removed by soaking it off in a bucket of warm water immediately. If there is discomfort some plasters can be removed with strong scissors, if parents cannot persevere with continuation of their use.

Chapter 10
Therapeutic Group Work

The child's need for group activities has long been recognized in the habilitation of handicapped children. Motor handicapped children are often isolated from their peers. They may not be able to run up and join a group of children, put an arm round a friend or even push away an annoying child. Parents find it difficult to bring the handicapped child into contact with other children whether normal or handicapped. Children need group treatment for contact with other children, sharing an activity with others, feeling part of a group and responding to competition and cooperation. Group work in therapy as well as in education offers opportunities for the child's social and emotional development.

Groups have been used in a variety of ways:

- *In speech therapy* for stimulation of communication and development of speech and language.
- *In occupational therapy* for perceptual training, for play involving perceptual motor function, for recreation, social interaction and learning to play a game involving rules and taking turns, and so on.
- *In physiotherapy* for training children with a specific diagnosis to carry out a set of exercises, for games involving gross motor activity, for swimming and activities in water, and various sports for the disabled.

As the aims of these different therapy groups overlap it is possible to carry out *interdisciplinary groups* of two kinds:

Playgroups including toy libraries, adventure playgrounds, special nursery schools, opportunity groups or nurseries, are orientated to each child's developmental levels and special problems. The therapists may advise or themselves work in the group setting, stimulating a few or occasionally all the children with play activities which involve gross motor, fine motor, perceptual and speech and language activities. The therapist may be in the playroom or nursery, relating to one child with specific problems and may or may not also bring in other children in the same activity.

The children may all be in the same room and may or may not feel themselves to belong to the same group in all activities.

Songs, storytime, percussion band, games and music may be the only sessions when all the children carry out the same activity. Therapists are also working with teachers, psychologists, child care staff, nursery nurses, nurses and parents in the therapeutic play groups.

The structured group works to treat or train a specific area of function. These groups integrate the gross motor, fine motor, perceptual, speech and language activities, but with more focus on any one of these areas. This focus may be on the major disability of the children in the group, say motor problems in cerebral palsied children. The focus may be on a specific area of function in one group session, whereas the focus will be on another area for that same group in other group sessions.

These structured interdisciplinary groups in Britain have been influenced by the ideas of Petö, Hari, and the work of physiotherapists Ester Cotton (1965, 1968, 1970, 1974, 1975), Dorothy Seglow, Monica Brewer and others who introduced these ideas in Britain. Many more Petö groups based on conductive education have developed in various parts of Britain (Hari & Tillemans 1984; Cottam & Sutton 1988; Hari & Akos 1990). Information can be obtained from SCOPE (The Spastics Society), London.

These groups may not follow the full system of the Petö approach, which involves very much more than a group session or group sessions. From studies with the staff of The Cheyne Centre for Children with Cerebral Palsy these structured interdisciplinary group sessions for multiply handicapped children were invaluable and often essential for such children (1969–1979).

Some of the main observations are:

(1) Individual sessions sometimes create too much pressure on the handicapped child and aggravate the normal or abnormal rebelliousness in a child. In the group such children often cooperate because all the other children present are doing what is expected of them.

(2) The one-to-one relationship in individual treatment may be too similar to the one-to-one relationship in the mother–child situation. This is normal in children under 3-year developmental level. Children with physical disabilities, however, are often over this age and need to relate to their peers *even though* their physical function may still be under a 3-year developmental level.

Although a child may need some private tuition in his school life and some disadvantaged children and children with very severe learning disabilities may still need this one-to-one relationship, many more need to 'grow out' of it emotionally and socially. Perhaps some of those who refuse to cooperate may be protesting at the dependency felt on being handled by the therapists all the time in this one-to-one situation.

(3) In the group, children follow instructions and imitate the other

children. Imitation helps the children with partial hearing loss or learning disability to understand what is required of them. In addition, the children in groups are observed to instruct and help each other carry out the programme of work.

(4) Speech is stimulated as the adult's concentration on all the children seems to take off the *pressure* on one child to speak.

(5) Concentration of the children who are working at their own pace is great. The attention span is far longer than in individual sessions; children work hard in groups lasting one and a half hours whilst in individual treatment for only 20–40 minutes.

(6) The programme consists of integrating aspects of physiotherapy, occupational therapy, speech therapy together with group work. It is planned by the team but carried out by one therapist and one or two aids or assistants. In this way a number of children are helped at the same time with economy on staff and on time spent getting children to and from each therapy department, as well as on time required to establish rapport with each different professional.

(7) Physiotherapists, occupational therapists, speech therapists, teachers, and nursery nurses welcome interdisciplinary groups as they can then see the total child and the relationship of their speciality to those of the others in his total function. On planning and using the structured group session the different disciplines are enabled to share their knowledge with one another so that practical integrated group activities can be created. Different disciplines have then to clarify their main aims with each child and make certain they are understood by everyone in the planning of the programme and in its execution. It is not possible for each professional to convey all her expertise to the other different disciplines, but rather to learn how to discover the overlap of her particular discipline with others. In this way the overlap becomes a practical achievement and enriches the teamwork.

General management of groups

Number of children   This varies according to the numbers of children in each centre, school or institution, from whom selections may be made. No matter how many children are in a group, they must be *involved* and preferably participating.

Staff   One staff member leads the group with another assisting her. The assistant should be from another discipline. If the children are all severely disabled, more help may be indicated. However, the adults present must be kept to a minimum, or their one-to-child relationship rather than a child-to-child relationship may occur. The leader may alternate with her assistant each week or alternate days in conducting the group.

All assistants need to work according to the leader's action and not divert the child's attention away from the group by private conversation with them or with each other.

Venue The group is best done in the child's own classroom or where there are no unfamiliar distractions and a coming and going of adults or other children.

Arrange children during the group session so that they can see the leader of the group at all times, and also so that the children see each other. Semi-circles or L-shaped seating arrangements are best, but the positions will change in a class with particular motor activities and mobility exercises.

Length of sessions should be planned for 1 to 2 hours depending on the children's ability to continue participating, and the programme of work.

Frequency Group sessions are best done daily or three times a week depending on the aims of the group programme. Some aims only require twice a week. The main object is that the children work together for not less than three times a week so that they know each other and develop a group dynamic.

Behaviour If a child refuses to join in, make sure that the programme is not too difficult for him. If it is not, let him watch for a while, ignoring him. The other children may be given a particularly pleasant activity or they may occasionally be told 'let's do that again for so-and-so to try as well'. Other ideas may be offered by the parent or team members who know the child. However, if non-participation continues or if the child seems oblivious to other children and cannot imitate others, the group cannot 'carry' him indefinitely. He may not be ready or not suitable for group treatments, and this is not always obvious in the beginning.

Children with behaviour problems may become disruptive to the group. Hyperkinetic children may be particularly difficult. However, try a trial period of partial sessions with the group, increase to full sessions and the techniques above. Restless children may settle down and join in with the others. Finally, good selection of children and programme planning makes organized management easier.

Selection of children

The basis for selection varies and ideas are still developing. The early days of group treatment both for staff and children seem to be easier if the disparity between the children is not great. A group with children who have hemiplegia and are at the walking level and at approximately the same chronological age and have intelligence form a group which works well. Such a group is best for inexperienced staff and for those professionals beginning group work. The hemiplegic group might enlarge itself to encompass other diagnostic types of cerebral palsy who have asymmetry. Mental levels of children may be varied. A variety of developmental levels among motor developmentally delayed children may be contained in one group. The following points influencing selection may be helpful.

Problems of children

MOTOR PROBLEMS

Selection of children according to diagnosis is not usually helpful. Select the children according to their problems. Although it is difficult to generalize them, motor problems are usually some or all of the following:

(1) Head control – postural fixation, particularly in the upright position.
(2) Head and trunk in midline, symmetrical arm and leg postures.
(3) Head and trunk counterpoising so that arms and legs can move into various asymmetrical postures or movements.
(4) Grasp to hold on, and grasp and release.
(5) Corrective movements and postures for any recurring abnormal positions of any joints; e.g. in spastic or athetoid children, elbow flexion, shoulder retraction, hip extension or semiflexion, adduction, knee flexion, equinis feet.
(6) Form of locomotion.
(7) Ability to sit or stand.
(8) Ability to rise from the floor or from a chair.

It is possible, say, to have a *pre-sitting group* with a selection of motor activity building up to sitting, prone to hands and knees and weight bearing on feet with trunk support (see developmental channels in Appendix, 0–6 months level). It is possible to have a group on *sitting and prewalking* with activities taken from the channels of development of 6–12 months (Appendix) or an ambulant group, 12 months and over (Appendix). The motor abilities selected for training will depend on the children with these problems. It is obviously essential to have assessments of the problems. The other aspects of function in the child should be considered, although motor problems are primary.

AGE OF CHILD

Children should be around the same chronological age, as their developmental levels alone will offer a range of children. It is sometimes an unhappy situation if a large boy of 11 with a developmental level of, say, sitting equal to about 6–9 months normal level is in a group with 3-year-olds also at this developmental level.

MENTAL LEVEL

The mental level should not cross too wide a spectrum. Some prefer keeping intelligent children in one group whilst others find it useful to mix as the mentally impaired child will imitate the intelligent child in carrying out the motor activity or other activities which do not demand high intelligence. Intellectually disabled children may also be better at movement than, say, a severely physically handicapped, intelligent athetoid child, thus a balance is obtained in the work programme.

PERSONALITY AND BEHAVIOUR

Personality of the children is rarely a consideration unless a child is excessively disruptive and management ideas for behaviour fail (see above). A child's emotional and social stages of development influence whether he or she is suitable.

OTHER DISABILITIES

Deaf, partially sighted or blind children may find it more difficult to join a group if the focus is on the motor handicap. However, again some athetoid children with high frequency hearing loss and some spastic children with partial hearing have responded well to groups through imitation, lip reading and other visual clues, as well as the fact that a good group session focused on problems other than specific hearing problems. Children with profound intellectual impairment may be too oblivious of the group dynamics being used and remain in their own world, and be unsuitable for such group work.

It must be remembered that factors for selection are still being explored by those working with groups.

Whatever the basis for selection the 'answer' to the best way to select children finally rests on whether group programmes of work can be created by the staff and on the ability of the leader of the group to weld her group of children together, so that they work together and there is a group spirit.

The programme

(1) It is essential to have this prepared before the group commences.
(2) It can be modified once used and *must* be changed as the children change and progress.
(3) The group leader needs to have the programme in front of her so

that she does not delay and lose any group impetus and collaboration gained. She must know 'what comes next', to maintain group concentration.

(4) The programme should not be too long, but it is better to spend more time on each item. The items are after all only chosen because they are to be trained and repetition is needed.

(5) Occasionally, have an easy item already achieved, as well as items *just beyond the* capacity of the children. If the children experience a successful achievement this motivates them further.

(6) Use action songs to carry out motor activities for the children, as they use the same songs each time, their familiarity is often appreciated. For many children, the programme should contain familiar elements, either songs, the playleader, the room, the time of day or days of the week and the general outline. However, the activities must gradually develop and change and not remain so predictable that the children do not progress.

ITEMS OF THE PROGRAMME

The programme and its further modifications must be assessed and reassessed, not only by the group leader, but also together with the other professional workers in the centre. Ongoing consultations are necessary to make sure that the items selected for the children motivate *all* the children and that any child is not 'carried' as a non-participant for too long.

Select items from the treatment suggestions in the chapters on developmental training and the problems of deformity. Give preference to those items which do not depend on holding or handling the child or there may be too many adults required. The presence of many adults disrupts the growing child–child relationships in the group. Select items which are at first easy and become more difficult as the children develop in the group programme. In addition, such selected items may be used in groups to show some children ahead of the others. This motivates the others to work towards these higher levels, which they can observe in their peers. In this way the therapist can have children at different levels of motor development in one group. She must have items selected so that they *build up* a particular motor ability.

For example

All the children sit around a large table. Children at 3–6 months developmental level of sitting will have to lean their trunks against the table and grasp a horizontal bar attached to the table or grasp a slatted table. The children from 6–9 months level do not lean against the table, but only grasp the support and the children from 9–12 months level who can sit alone, do so with their hands at their sides or on their laps.

Similarly, standing may be modified from standing leaning against the table with grasp support, stand and grasp, and stand alone.

Also prone lying raise head, prone lying raise head and rise on to elbows, and prone lying raise head and rise on to hands can be included simultaneously. With careful planning and assessment of the children many more examples will be found.

All motor activities must be associated with perceptual experience of direction, spatial relationships, colour, body awareness, various matching activities in relating shapes, sizes, textures as well as speech and language, social awareness and of course the fun of children working and playing together (Fig. 10.1).

Music and movement, songs, action songs, fingerplays and any other children's songs and music must be used for group work. However, as with the other activities, these must be modified to relate to the children's levels of development and interest. Imaginative activities such as 'pretend you are a tree in the wind' or 'let's wave our arms like birds' which are used for children's groups should not be used unless the children understand them and are at the 'let's pretend' level of play development. This is about the 3 year level.

Children's group games and party games may also be adapted and used in group work. Whatever items are selected they *must not* be random, but selected according to aims of therapy with each child. There will be aims of therapy which cannot be realized in the group sessions, or not enough in the group sessions. *Individual sessions* will be necessary for the children. However, if the child is well selected and the items well chosen for him in the group, individual sessions may not be essential for him, for a period.

It is not possible to give programmes for groups as these must be

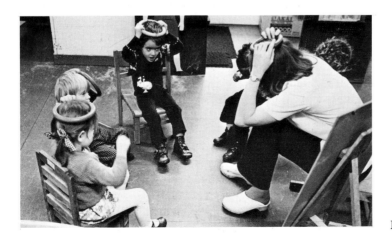

Fig 10.1

composed around the children themselves. However, the following should be included:

(1)   Start and end with a dressing activity, e.g. taking shoes and socks off, or taking a cardigan off.
(2)   Fetch and put away any equipment for the group.
(3)   Use gross motor activities for one session, integrating this with perception and language activities.
(4)   Use hand classes for a session, integrating this with perception and language activities.
(5)   Have a meal or tea for the group in order to include feeding training and washing hands.
(6)   Suggested group games for walkers and non-walkers. These may include crawling hand ball, passing ball or objects in sitting, throwing beanbags into large containers, obstacle course, croquet, ring toss, deck quoits, carpet bowls, shuffle board, rolling balls on the table or floor, ping-pong with the ball attached to a high horizontal wire for ball retrieval and other play activities. Board games should have large counters or handles on the draught pieces or holes for the pieces and other adaptations.

Summary

Interdisciplinary group work is valuable in the treatment of cerebral palsied and motor delayed children. They require consultations between staff:

(1)   To assess children's functions in all areas before and *during* group sessions.
(2)   To plan, monitor and progress the items of the group programmes.

It is best for one person to carry out the programme with perhaps other professionals occasionally assisting but *not* interrupting during the group session itself. Adjustments of the programme can be discussed after the session is over.

Teachers and therapists depend on each other to create dynamic group sessions and therefore must work closely together.

Appendix 1
Developmental Levels

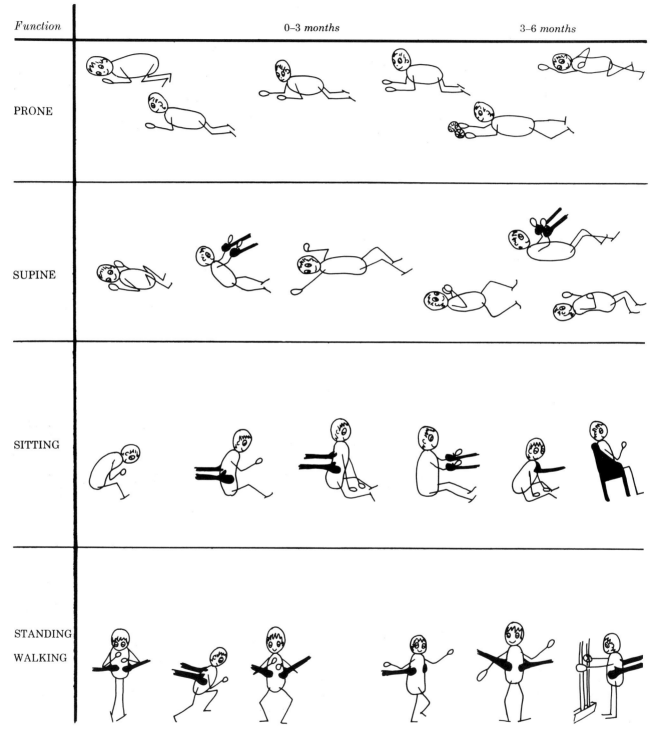

6–9 *months*   9–12 *months*

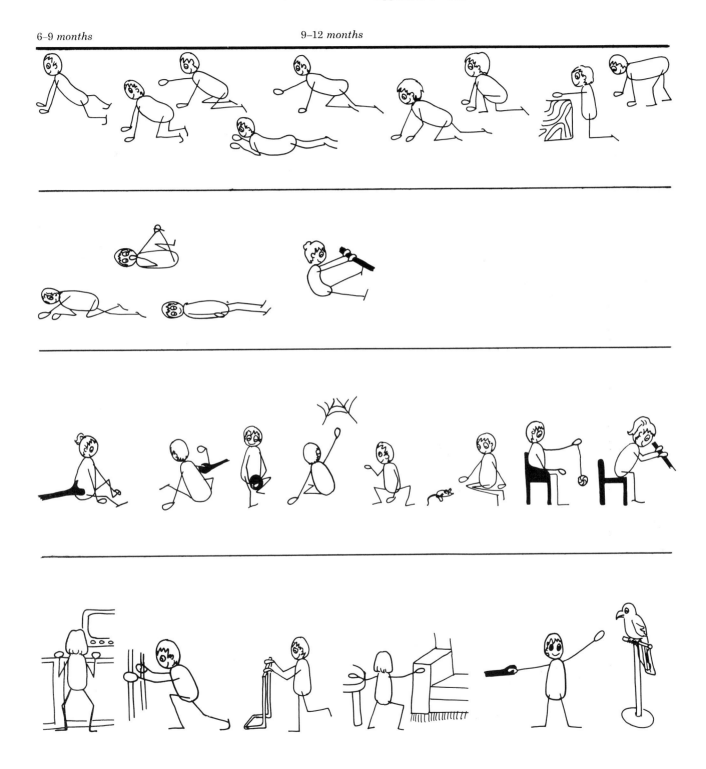

Physical ability assessment guide

Scoring key

0 – No ability, no initiation
1 – Initiates alone
2 – Partial, laboured, unreliable or infrequent
3 – Completes alone reliably but very abnormal performance
4 – Completes reliably with near normal/normal performance

Maintains posture – 10 seconds
Locomotion – 10 steps
Stairs – 4 steps

Prone

0–3 months	Can be placed, head turns
	Raises head up
	Maintains head up
	On forearms, head, chest up
	Rises on to knees and forearms
3–6 months	Reaches forward with right arm (extended)
	Reaches forward with left arm (extended)
	Rolls over to right
	Rolls over to left
6–9 months	Creeps on abdomen
	Maintains on hands, elbows straight
	Rises on to hands and knees
	Maintains hands and knees
	Reaches forward with one hand, on hands posture
9–12 months	On hands and knees, lifts arm and opposite leg
	Pivots body using limbs to right
	Pivots body using limbs to left
	Crawls reciprocally
	Achieves sit from hands and knees
	Half-kneels with hand supports
	Rises to upright kneeling with hand supports
	Walks on hands and feet
12–24 months	Creeps on to table/couch
	Crawls upstairs
	Crawls downstairs backwards
	Kneels upright, hips straight, no support
	Half-kneels upright, no support
	Knee walks forwards
	Rises to stand, no support

Supine

0–3 months	Can be placed, head turns
	Head lag overcome slightly
	Reaches out along floor, to side
3–6 months	Head maintained in midline, symmetrical weight bears
	Hands together, symmetry
	Head raises, head lag overcome
	Reaches up, across body
	Bridges hips into extension, feet flat
6–9 months	Rolls over to right
	Rolls over to left
	Reaches, grasps foot
	Lying straight, arms down, head midline, turns
9–12 months	Rises to sitting through right side-lying, alone
	Rises to sitting through left side-lying, alone
	Pulls self to sitting

Sitting

0–3 months	Can be placed, head, trunk supported, flexes, hips
	Vertical head control, trunk supported
	Leans on forearms or hands, trunk supported
3–6 months	Sits leaning on hands, no support to trunk
	Sits in chair with back, sides or chest support
6–9 months	Sits with one hand support, uses other hand
	Saves self on hands forwards
	Sits arms free, alone
	Saves self to right side
	Saves self to left side
	Sits leaning forwards, re-erects alone
9–12 months	Sits, reaches across, to side, above head
	Sits and turns, reaches to right
	Sits and turns, reaches to left
	Side-sits on right hip
	Side-sits on left hip
	Changes to hands and knees
	Sits alone on regular chair
	Sits on chair, reaches in all directions
	Rises from sit to standing, holding on
	Sits and pivots on floor
	Sits and pivots on chair
	Bottom shuffles along floor
	Tilt reactions anterior-posterior
	Tilt reactions laterally

12–18 months	Seats self on low stool
	Rises from sit to stand, no holding
	Sits on high stool, legs dangling
	Squats at play
	Squat rises to stand and returns to squat
	Saves self if tipped backwards

Stand and walk

0–6 months	Weight bears, plantigrade feet, trunk support
	Steps, trunk supported
6–9 months	Stands, forearm leaning or holding on, pelvis supported
	Stands, holds on alone, hips may flex, feet flat
9–12 months	Pulls self to standing, holds on
	Stands, holds on, lifts right leg
	Stands, holds on, lifts left leg
	Cruises using two hands
	Stands, holds one hand, reaches in all directions
12–18 months	Stands alone
	Stands stoop and recover
	Walks, two hands held or grasps walker
	Walks, one hand held
	Walks alone
	Walks, carrying object
	Rises to stand from all positions, no support
	Walks backwards
	Walks upstairs, holds both sides, two feet per step
	Protective stagger reaction if pushed sideways
	Protective stagger reaction if pushed forward
	Protective stagger reaction if pushed backward
18–24 months	Stands, kicks ball
	Throws ball overhead
	Runs
	Walks, stops and turns (pivot)
	Walks upstairs, holding one rail, two feet per step
	Walks downstairs, both rails, two feet per step
2–3 years	Jumps in place
	Jumps off 6 inch step
	Pedals tricycle
	Broad jump (8 inches)
	Walks downstairs, one rail, alternate feet
	Walks upstairs, no hold, alternate feet
	Walks downstairs, no hold, alternate feet
3–4 years	Stands on preferred leg (5–10 seconds)
	Hops on preferred leg
	Heel-to-toe walk

	Catches bounced ball

Catches bounced ball
Uses large bat
4–5 years   Balances on one leg, 10 seconds
Walks on narrow, straight line
Walks between 8 inch parallels
Walks on narrow plank/bench
Steps over knee-high stick with right
Steps over knee-high stick with left
Backward, heel-to-toe walk

Note:
- Ages are in approximate sequence.
- Select items in each section (prone, supine, sit, stand) as aims/objectives in a developmental therapy plan.
- Record items achieved with dates; use scoring key for outcomes/evaluations.
- All gross motor items from the Denver developmental screening test are included and based on those ages.
- This guide is similar to the gross motor function measure which was validated as responsive to changes in child's function with inter-rater and intra-rater reliability (see Russe *et al.* 1989).

Wheelchair use
Development of abilities – assessment outline:

Sits upright in wheelchair
Finds and grasps wheel on right side
Finds and grasps wheel on left side
Grasps both wheels simultaneously
Moves right wheel forward slightly (2 inches)
Moves left wheel forward slightly (2 inches)
Moves right wheel forward over 1 foot
Moves left wheel forward over 1 foot
Moves both wheels forward over 1 foot
Moves right wheel backward
Moves left wheel backward
Moves both wheels backward
Travels forward, brings wheelchair to a halt
Travels backward, brings wheelchair to a halt
Starts from stationary, turns wheelchair to right, 180°
Starts from stationary, turns wheelchair to left, 180°
Propels wheelchair round obstacles
Propels wheelchair between two objects forward
Propels wheelchair between two objects backward

- Increase distances and speed
- Explore child's own strategies

Transfers
Sitting, uses brake to halt wheelchair
Sitting, lifts leg rests out of way
Sit slides forward in seat pushing on arm rests
Sit slides forward in seat using semipivot pelvis
Sit rises to stand on plantigrade feet, uses arm rests or
Sit rises to stand, uses arms forward to grasp support
Sit transfers laterally to bed, to toilet, to chair
Sit slides along transfer board to new seat, uses hand
Sit transfers out of seat downward, to kneel or sit
Sit rises to stand using arm rests or grasping support
Sit to stand, changes to new seat
Repeats any of the above in safe return to wheelchair

- Modify this list according to each child's own strategy and condition
- Therapist uses physical guidance and support to teach
- Demonstrate transfers to parents *and* carers so that they bend hips and knees correctly, and protect their own backs

Appendix 2
Equipment

Selection of equipment

Selection and provision of equipment should always be supervised by each child's therapists and medical specialists.

Select equipment according to the following considerations.

(1) *Assessment of the child's disabilities and abilities*, especially emerging 'unreliable' abilities. The correct amount of aid makes it possible for him to carry out tasks otherwise impossible, but too much aid prevents his own participation and development of emerging ability.

(2) *Assessment of the child's deformities* or threatening deformities. Good alignment in any apparatus and correction of abnormal postures must be maintained during the use of the equipment. For example, standing may be correct in a standing box, but become abnormal on hand function in standing; sitting may be upright in a push-chair with special modifications but become abnormal when the chair is pushed by an adult!

(3) *Good design* of equipment takes account of adjustments for child's growth, removal of supports with increasing ability, a variety of modifications for different children in a clinic/school, is as portable as possible and looks as normal as possible. Simple designs easily adjusted by busy parents and staff are desirable.

(4) Equipment provides a variety of additional motor experiences in different positions. It offers children appropriate support so that they can participate in social and educational activities.

(5) Use different items of equipment for a variety of postures through-out the day as part of the prevention and correction of deformities. Check positioning at night and turn child. Equipment at night may interfere with sleeping patterns of a child.

Ongoing supervision is important to check the following:

(1) *Measurements* of the child as he grows so that equipment is not too small.

(2) *Value of the equipment* in relation to achievements gained in therapy and daily care. Once again equipment must facilitate independence, not substitute for it.

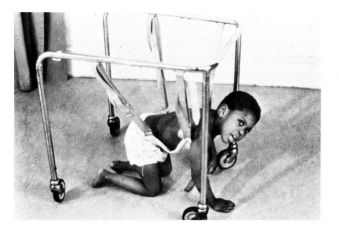

Fig. 1 A crawler.

casters is essentially the basic principle used in crawlers (Fig.1). Many adjustments may be required, e.g. straps to hold the thighs in flexion and prevent *shooting* into abnormal extension; straps to stop thighs or arms pushing into the area beneath the child's abdomen; small wedge, straps or cushion to stop child sliding off crawler and adjustments of the height of the body support so that the length of the child's arms reaches the distance to the floor from that abdominal–chest support. Platforms on wheels, wedges on wheels (casters) or toy creations such as the dolphin on casters are also used by some children for crawling on hands only, on knees only, or on hands and knees.

Apparatus for supported standing   Various standing frames are available (Fig. 2). The child can stand and hold parallel or vertical bars; backs of chairs or stationary walking aids.

Note   Standing aids do not train standing unless the aid is vertical with the line of gravity going from the child's head (ear) down to just behind his ankle. Adjust the foot pieces of the skis or straps of the stabilizer (standing frame to thigh or to knee) to obtain the correct alignment. Any aid with a forward or a backward lean is of value to correct flexed hips by strapping (knees by knee pieces and feet held at right angles by a board and/or foot pieces).

Prone boards/forward standing frame attached at a forward angle to a table for schoolwork or hand activities corrects abnormal postures of the legs, keeps the trunk straight and stimulates head control and arm function. Standing boards on tilt-frames do the same and are used more for ball throwing, arm exercises and periods of passive stretching of flexors and plantar flexors. Large pommels or other ideas may be incorporated

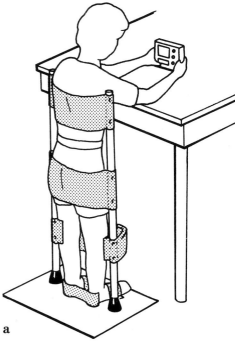

a

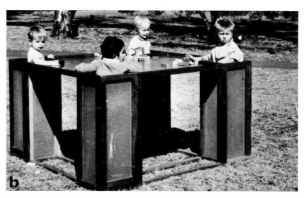

b

b

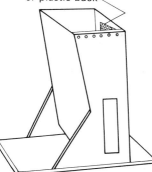

See-through mesh
or plastic back

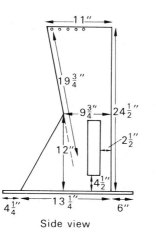

c

Side view

Fig. 2 a, Standing frame, supporting chest, hips, knees and feet. b, Standing table. Backs of standing boxes can be of wire mesh to observe leg postures. Note lower level of dark-haired child to encourage arm reach and counteract adducted-flexed spastic arms. c, Standing box. There is a foot platform which can be fitted in to make the standing box adaptable for a smaller child. A 'V'-shaped wedge on the platform keeps the child's feet in a good position. A ledge is attached to both sides of the box and the bars of the tray are made to slide over this. The tray is slid on and fixed in position with bolts fitting into holes on the side of the box. These holes and wire mesh at the back enable the therapist to see the child is in a good position. The rim of the tray is about $\frac{3}{4}$ inch (18.7 mm) high. (*Note* 1 inch = 25 mm.)

to keep legs apart and also occasionally externally rotated. None of these aids train standing but give correct postures and prevent deformity.

Walking aids There are a great variety and they should be carefully selected (see Figs 7.177–7.179).

- *With trunk support* given by a padded support to chest or by chest slings attached overhead.
- *Without trunk support.* A four point walker which can be pushed with grasp on the sides of the child or grasp in front of the child (see Fig. 7.177). Toy walkers or doll's prams are very popular. Large soft toys on wheels, large trucks, large toy boxes on casters and similar normal toys should be stable, weighted and checked for size according to the child. Pushing stable children's or adult's chairs which slide easily but not too quickly as well as boxes on skis and other simple aids also train walking.

    Note Check that wheels on walkers are correct for the child. If they 'run away', preventing correct postures and establishment of the child's own control of his balance, use the walkers with crutch tips at each of the four points, ski sliders or other modifications. Various walkers without wheels are on the market. Crutches, elbow crutches, quadripods, tripods and thick based sticks are used for *selected* children (Fig. 3). Frequently progress is made from crutches to sticks. Check length, hand grasps and stability. Some sticks (of wood) may be linked together with a centre piece for initial stability.

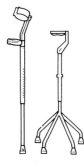
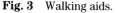

Fig. 3 Walking aids.

Note All walking aids should be checked for height so that the child does not grasp them with abnormal shoulder hunching, excessive flexion of the elbows and radial deviation of wrists. If grasp is not possible without these abnormalities try a walking aid which requires pushing with flat hands and straight elbows, or use a chair.

Parallel bars These should be adjustable in height, sometimes in width. Hand slides are used if the child cannot grasp and release to use the parallel bars. A chair at the end of the bars may be used for training standing up from sitting. Eversion boards, foot prints and abduction boards have been placed between the bars when needed. Do not use parallel bars for spastics who grasp in excessive flexion which cannot be eliminated by lowering the bars for elbow extension.

Appliances for correct posture in standing; weight bearing; trunk control, and to *weight* the feet of unstable athetoids or ataxics with below-knee appliances:

- *Long leg calipers* (braces) which have thigh bands, knee pieces and fit into boots. These keep knees straight. Knees may unlock to allow sitting. There may be pelvic bands and adjustments to lock/unlock hip to keep hips straight and facing forward, with some abduction. Abduction-external rotation is not often possible in spasticity. A rotator coil may help, but could twist the knee too much. Also, T-straps and back or front locks attached to the long leg brace at the ankle (see below-knee iron).

- *Below-knee irons* with attachment to the heel of the child's boot, under the heel or having a joint opposite the ankle. The iron locks against a stop to prevent plantarflexion (back stop) or to prevent dorsiflexion (front stop). T-strap inside to counter pronation. T-strap outside to counter varus. Foot or heel moulds may be inserted inside the boots for arch supports, inner side, to control valgus. Ankle-foot orthoses with trainers or boots (Figs 9.11 and 9.12). Orthoses are more corrective than below-knee irons and keep the calcaneous in a better neutral position.

- *Knee gaiters* or polythene knee moulds, plaster knee moulds to keep knees straight (Fig. 4).
- *Abduction pants* to keep legs apart. It may need stiffening with some light plastic material if adduction is strong (Fig. 5).
- *Elbow gaiters* which keep elbows straight for correct arm push and grasp of walkers and other poles in other functions (Fig. 6).

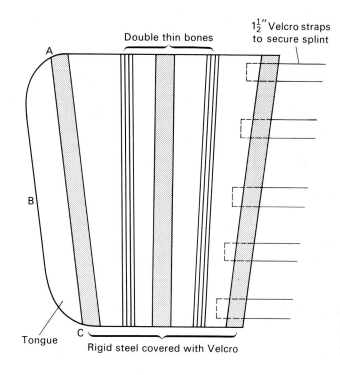

Fig. 4 Leg gaiter made of white coutil. It is wrapped around the leg bringing Velcro straps over the front side of 'B'.

FEEDING

Dycem mat, long-handled spoons, spoons of different sizes, metal and unbreakable plastic spoons, rubberzote and other handles, dishes with and without sides. Suction rubbers to hold bowl on table. Bibs. Cups; non-slip, weighted, sponge rubber suctions to hold cup and straw steady; baby mugs with non-spill aids and training lids with small opening. Mugs with two handles and one handle which is easy to grasp.

DRESSING

Velcro. Zips and special designs. Detachable fronts for children who drool or mess. Large buttons, hooks or other fastenings.

BATHING

Non-slip mat in bath, small bath within large bath. Inflatable chair propped in bath, neck supports, bath seats hooked on sides. Liquid bath cleansers to avoid soaping when there are difficulties.

TOILET

See sections on chairs and sitting and Figs 7.125–7.127.

SLEEPING BAGS, COTS, BABY TOYS, ETC.

As for normal babies.

PRAMS, PUSHCHAIRS AND BABY BUGGIES

As for normal children but check postures more carefully. Special inserts and buggies which correct posture are available on the market.

WHEELCHAIRS

A variety are available. References should be made to manufacturers of medical equipment, departments of health and voluntary organizations as lists of wheelchairs and their designs change and improve (see list of organizations above, in particular the Disabled Living Foundation, and Wheelchair use in the Appendix). The principles of correct sitting discussed in Chapter 7 on the development of sitting and chairs should be applied to the child in wheelchairs with the added considerations:

(1) Can he propel the chair himself or must it be pushed? Can he transfer?
(2) Facilities of the child's home for containing a wheelchair – stairs,

doorways, sizes of rooms, use of table heights available, etc.
(3)   Is the wheelchair useful indoors, outdoors or both?
(4)   Can the wheelchair 'grow' with the child. What modifications?
(5)   Can the wheelchair be transported, stored, put on public transport?

Contact Communication Aids Centres for electronic devices.

SPECIAL AIDS IN THE CLASSROOM

Typewriters; electronic aids to communication (augmented communication aids and also called communication systems). Advice and professional skills can be obtained from communication advice centres, The Wolfson Centre, The Cheyne Centre for Children with Cerebral Palsy and others. Contact: ISAAC (International Society for Augmentative and Alternative Communication), Centre for Human Communication, Oak

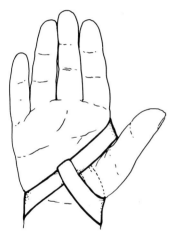

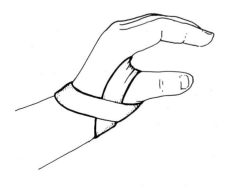

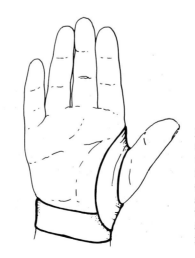

Fig. 7   Thumb splint to correct adducted-flexed thumb. A cock-up wrist splint to midline may be incorporated if palm flexion is excessive. Figure of eight thumb splint at base of thumb and over the wrist in soft pigskin or simply a handkerchief may be adequate for babies and young children.

Tree Lane, Selly Oak, Birmingham, B29 6SA. Various aids such as page-turners, pencil holders, page and book holders, various clips for drawing/ writing paper and special low vision aids are among many classroom aids offered by manufacturers of medical and educational equipment in their lists. Occupational therapists should be consulted.

AIDS TO MOBILITY

Aids other than walkers, crawlers and wheelchairs such as go-karts, Chailey chariots; tricycles with adaptations. Hand-propelled tricycles. Prone tricycles. Corner seat on casters. A variety of mobility toys is in development by engineers, research workers, parents, therapists and toy manufacturers. See Adventure Playground organizations and the Disabled Living Foundation, above.

Many toys and mobility aids are now operated by a variety of switches for severely impaired people. Enquire to Occupational Therapy and Speech Therapy organizations about these electronic devices.

GENERAL

Helmets to protect the child's head if he falls frequently. Toy catalogues. Toy libraries' catalogues for appropriate toys. Gym apparatus (balls, hoops, ropes, climbing apparatus). Adventure playground apparatus, play-things and equipment. Rocking boards, rocking toys, swings, slides, climbing frames. Thumb splints (Fig. 7). Wrist, hand and thumb splints are tailor made for each child.

Note Treatment tables in physiotherapy should be high for some physiotherapy techniques and low for training the child to get off the treatment table into standing, to climb, etc.

References

Andre-Thomas, C.S., St Anne Dargassies, S. & Chesni, Y. (1960) *Neurological Examination of the Infant*. Heinemann – Spastic International Medical Publications, London.

Ayres, A.J. (1979) *Sensory Integration and the Child*. Western Psychological Services, Los Angeles.

Bailey, D.B. & Simeonsson, R.J. (1988) *Family Assessment in Early Intervention*. Merrill, Columbus, Ohio.

Bailey, D.B., Simeonsson, R.J., Buysse, V. & Smith, T. (1993) Reliability of an index of child characteristics. *Dev. Med. Child Neurol.*, **35**, 806.

Bairstow, P., Cochrane, R. & Hur, J. (1993) Shortened version: *Evaluation of Conductive Education for Children with Cerebral Palsy (Final Report)*. HMSO, London.

Bairstow, P., Cochrane, R. & Rusk, I. (1991) Selection of children with cerebral palsy for conductive education. *Dev. Med. Child Neurol.*, **33**, 984.

Bardsley, D.G.I. (1993) Seating. In *Elements of Paediatric Physiotherapy* (ed. P. Eckersley). Churchill Livingstone, Edinburgh.

Bax, M.C.O. (1964) Terminology and classification of cerebral palsy. *Dev. Med. Child Neurol.*, **6**, 295.

Beach, R.C. (1988) Conductive education for motor disorders: new hope or false hope. *Arch. Dis. Child.*, **63**, 211.

Belenkii, V.Y., Gurfinkel, V.S. & Paltsev, Y.I. (1967) Elements of control of voluntary movements. *Biophysics*, **12**, 135.

Bleck, E.E. (1987) *Orthopaedic Management in Cerebral Palsy. Clin. Dev. Med.* No. 99/100, MacKeith Press, Blackwell Scientific Publications, Oxford.

Blencowe, S.M. (ed.) (1969) *Cerebral Palsy and the Young Child*. Livingstone, London.

Bobath, B. (1965) *Abnormal Postural Reflex Activity Caused by Brain Lesions*. Heinemann, London.

Bobath, B. (1967) The very early treatment of cerebral palsy. *Dev. Med. Child Neurol.*, **9**(4), 373.

Bobath, B. (1971) Motor development, its effect on general development and application to the treatment of cerebral palsy. *Physiotherapy*, **57**, 526.

Bobath, B. & Bobath, K. (1975) *Motor Development in the Different Types of Cerebral Palsy*. Heinemann, London.

Bobath, K. (1971) The normal postural reflex mechanism and its deviation in children with cerebral palsy. *Physiotherapy*, **57**, 515.

Bobath, K. (1980) *A Neurophysiological Basis for the Treatment of Cerebral Palsy. Clin. Dev. Med.* No. 75, SIMP, Heinemann Medical, London.

Bobath, K. & Bobath, B. (1972) Cerebral palsy, part 1, and the neurodevelopmental approach to treatment, part 2. In *Physical Therapy Services in the Developmental Disabilities* (eds P.H. Pearson & C.E. Williams). C.C. Thomas, Springfield, Illinois.

Bobath, K. & Bobath, B. (1984) The neuro-developmental treatment. In *Management of the Motor Disorders of Children with Cerebral Palsy* (ed. D. Scrutton),

p. 6. SIMP, Blackwell Scientific Publications Oxford.

Bower, E. & McLellan, D.L. (1992) Effect of increased exposure to physiotherapy on skill acquisition of children with cerebral palsy. *Dev. Med. Child Neurol.*, **34**, 25.

Bowley, A.H. & Gardiner, L. (1969) *The Young Handicapped Child*. Livingstone, London.

Brazelton, T. (1976) Case finding, screening, diagnosis and tracking. Discussants' comments. In *Intervention Strategies for High Risk Infants and Grandchildren* (ed. T.D. Tjossem). University Park Press, Baltimore.

Brereton, B. (1971) *Learning Ability*. The Spastics Centre, NSW, Australia.

Brereton, B. & Sattler, J. (1975) *Cerebral Palsy: Basic Abilities*, 2nd edn. The Spastics Centre of New South Wales, Sydney, Australia.

Brunnstrom, S. (1970) *Movement Therapy in Hemiplegia – A Neurophysiological Approach*. Harper & Row, New York.

Burns, Y. (1970) Reduction of hypertonicity with the use of plasters. *Aust. J. Physiother*, **XVL**, 3 September.

Butler, P.B. & Nene, A.V. (1991) The biomechanics of fixed ankle-foot orthoses and their potential in the management of cerebral palsied children. *Physiotherapy*, **77**, 81.

Butler, P.B., Thompson, N. & Major, R.E. (1992) Improvement in walking performance of children with cerebral palsy (preliminary results). *Dev. Med. Child Neurol.*, **34**, 567.

Campbell, S.K. (ed.) (1991) *Pediatric Neurologic Physical Therapy*, 2nd edn. Churchill Livingstone, New York.

Capute, A.J., Accordo, P.J., Vining, E.P.G., Rubenstein, J.E. & Harryman, S. (1978) Primitive reflex profile. *Monographs in Developmental Pediatrics*, Vol. 1. University Park Press, Baltimore.

Capute, A.J., Palmer, F.B., Shapiro, B.K., Wachtel, R.C., Ross, A. & Accordo, P.J. (1984) Primitive reflex profile: a quantitation of primitive reflexes in infancy. *Dev. Med. Child Neurol.*, **26**, 375.

Carlsen, P.N. (1975) Comparison of two occupational therapy approaches for treating the young cerebral-palsied child. *Am. J. Occup. Ther.*, **29**, 267.

Carr, J.H., Shepherd, R.B. (1987) A motor learning model for rehabilitation. In *Movement Science: Foundations for Physical Therapy in Rehabilitation* (eds J.H. Carr & R.B. Shepherd), p. 31. Aspen, Rockville, Maryland.

Chiou, I.L. & Burnett, C.N. (1985) Values of activities of daily living. *Phys. Ther.*, **65**, 901.

Cioni, G., Ferrari, F. & Prechtl, H.F.R. (1989) Posture and spontaneous motility in fullterm infants. *Early Human Dev.*, **18**, 247.

Cioni, G., Ferrari, F. & Prechtl, H.F.R. (1992) Early motor assessment in brain-damaged preterm infants. In *Movement Disorders in Children* (eds H. Forssberg & H. Hirschfeld), p. 72. Karger, Basel.

Collins, J. & Brinkworth, R. (1973) *Improving Babies with Down's Syndrome*, 5th edn. N.I. Region, National Society for Mentally Handicapped Children, Annadale Ave., Belfast.

Collis, E. (1947) *A Way of Life for the Handicapped Child*. Faber & Faber, London.

Collis, E. (1953) Management of cerebral palsy in children. *Med. Illustr.*, **7**.

Collis, E., Collis, R., Dunham, W., Hilliard, L.T. & Lawson, D. (1956) *The Infantile Cerebral Palsies*. Heinemann, London.

Cooper, J., Moodley, M. & Reynell, J. (1978) *Helping Language Development*. Edward Arnold, London.

Cordo, P.J. & Nashner, L.M. (1982) Properties of postural adjustments associated with rapid arm movements. *J. Neurophysiol.*, **47**, 287.

Cottam, P. & Sutton, A. (1988) *Conductive Education: a System for Overcoming Motor Disorder*. Croom Helm, London.

Cotton, E. (1965) The Institute for Movement Therapy and School for Conductors, Budapest, Hungary. *Dev. Med. Child Neurol.*, **17**, 437.

Cotton, E. (1968) Conductive education with special reference to severe athetoids in a non-residential centre. *J. Ment. Subnorm.*, **14**(26), 50.

Cotton, E. (1970) Integration of treatment and education in cerebral palsy. *Physiotherapy*, **56**(4), 143.

Cotton, E. (1974) Improvement in Motor Function with the use of Conductive Education. *Dev. Med. Child Neurol.*, **16**, 637.

Cotton, E. (1975a) *The Basic Motor Pattern*. The Spastics Society, London.

Cotton, E. (1975b) *Conductive Education and Cerebral Palsy*. The Spastics Society, London.

Cratty, B.J. (1970) *Perceptual and Motor Development in Infants and Children*. Macmillan, London.

Cratty, B.J. (1969) *Perceptuo-Motor Efficiency in Children*. Lea & Febiger, Philadelphia.

Crothers, B. & Paine, R.S. (1959) *The Natural History of Cerebral Palsy*. Harvard University Press, Cambridge, Massachusetts.

Cummins, R.A. (1988) *The Neurologically Impaired Child: Doman-Delacato Techniques Reappraised*. Croom Helm, London.

Cusick, B. & Sussman, M. (1982) Short leg casts. Their role in the management of cerebral palsy. *Phys. Occup. Ther. Pediatr.*, **2**, 93.

Deaver, G.G. (1956) Cerebral palsy – methods of treating the neuromuscular disabilities. *Arch. Phys. Med.*, **37**, 363.

Decker, R. (1962) *Motor Integration*. Thomas, Springfield, Illinois.

Denhoff, E. (1967) *Cerebral Palsy – The Preschool Years*. Thomas, Springfield, Illinois.

Denhoff, E. & Robinault, I.P. (1960) *Cerebral Palsy and Related Disorders*. McGraw-Hill, New York.

Dietz, V. (1992) Spasticity: exaggerated reflexes or movement disorder? In *Movement Disorders in Children* (eds H. Forssberg & H. Hirschfeld), p. 225. Karger, Basel.

Dietz, V. & Berger, W. (1983) Normal and impaired regulation of muscle stiffness in gait: a new hypothesis about muscle hypertonia. *Exp. Neurol.*, **79**, 680.

Doman, G., Doman, R. *et al.* (1960) Children with severe brain injuries. Neurological organisation in terms of mobility. *JAMA*, **174**, 257.

Drillien, C.M. & Drummond, M.B. (eds) (1977) *Neurodevelopmental Problems in Early Childhood: Assessment and Management*. Blackwell Scientific, Oxford.

Drillien, C.M. & Drummond, M.B. (1983) *Developmental Screening and the Child with Special Needs*. Heinemann, London.

Dunn, C., Williams, V. & Young, C. (1990) *Guidelines for Good Practice*. Association of Paediatric Chartered Physiotherapists, c/o CSP, 14 Bedford Row, London WCIR 4ED.

Eckersley, P.M. (1990) Cerebral palsy and profound retardation. In *Profound Retardation and Multiple Impairment* (eds J. Hogg *et al.*). Chapman & Hall, London.

Eckersley, P.M. (ed.) (1993) *Elements of Paediatric Physiotherapy*. Churchill Livingstone, Edinburgh.

Edwards, S., Partridge, C.J. & Mee, R. (1990) Treatment schedules for research: a model for physiotherapy. *Physiotherapy*, **76**, 605.

Egan, D., Illingworth, R.S. & Mackeith, R.C. (1974) *Developmental Screening 0–5 years*. Heinemann – Spastics International Medical Publications, London.

Egel, P.F. (1948) *Technique of Treatment for the Cerebral Palsy Child*. C.V.

Mosby, St Louis, USA.

Ellenberg, J.H. & Nelson, K.B. (1981) Early recognition of infants at high risk for cerebral palsy: examination at age four months. *Dev. Med. Child Neurol.*, **23**, 705.

Farber, S.D. (1982) A multisensory approach to neurorehabilitation. In *Neurorehabilitation: A Multisensory Approach* (ed. S.D. Farber). Saunders, Philadelphia.

Fay, T. (1954a) Rehabilitation of patients with spastic paralysis. *J. Intern. Coll. Surgeons*, **22**, 200.

Fay, T. (1954b) Use of pathological and unlocking reflexes in the rehabilitation of spastics. *Am. J. Phys. Med.*, **33**(6), 347.

Featherstone, H. (1981) *A Difference in the Family*. Basic Books, New York.

Feldenkrais, M. (1980) *Awareness Through Movement*. Penguin Books, London.

Finnie, N. (1974) *Handling the Young Cerebral Palsied Child at Home*, 2nd edn. Heinemann, London.

Fiorentino, M. (1963) *Reflex Testing Methods for Evaluation of C.N.S. Development*. Thomas, Springfield, Illinois.

Fisher, A.G., Murray, E. & Bundy, A. (1991) *Sensory Integration: Theory and practice*. Davis, Philadelphia.

Foley, J. (1965) The treatment of cerebral palsy and allied disorders in the young child. In *Physical Medicine in Paediatrics* (ed. B. Kiernander). Butterworths, London.

Foley, J. (1977a) Cerebral palsy – physical aspects. In *Neurodevelopmental Problems in Early Childhood: Assessment and Management* (eds C.M. Drillien & M.B. Drummond), p. 269. Blackwell Scientific Publications, Oxford.

Foley, J. (1977b) Cerebral palsy – associated disorders. In *Neurodevelopmental Problems in Early Childhood: Assessment and Management* (eds C.M. Drillien & M.B. Drummond), p. 282. Blackwell Scientific Publications, Oxford.

Foley, J. (1983) The athetoid syndrome. *J. Neurol. Neurosurg. Psychiatry*, **46**, 289.

Forssberg, H. (1985) Ontogeny of human locomotor control I. Infant stepping, supported locomotion and transition to independent locomotion. *Exp. Brain Res.*, **57**, 480.

Forssberg, H. & Hirschfeld, H. (eds) (1992) *Movement Disorders in Children*. Karger, Basel.

Fox, A.M. (1975) *They Get This Training But They Don't Really Know How You Feel: Transcripts of Interviews with Parents of Handicapped Children*. Institute of Child Health, London.

Fraiberg, S. (1977) *Insights from the Blind*. Human Horizon Series. Souvenir Press (Educational and Academic), London.

French, J. & Patterson, M. (1992) Psychological development of the child: its implications for physiotherapy practice. In *Physiotherapy: A Psychosocial Approach* (ed. S. French). Butterworth-Heinemann, London.

Fulford, G.E. & Brown, J.K. (1976) Position as a cause of deformity in children with cerebral palsy. *Dev. Med. Child Neurol.*, **18**, 305.

Gentile, A.M. (1987) Skill acquisition: action, movement and neuromotor processes. In *Movement Science: Foundations for Physical Therapy in Rehabilitation* (eds J.H. Carr & R.B. Shepherd), p. 93. Aspen, Rockville, Maryland.

Gesell, A. (1971) *The First Five Years of Life*. Harper & Row, New York.

Gillette, H.E. (1969) *Systems of Therapy in Cerebral Palsy*. Thomas, Springfield, Illinois.

Giuliani, C.A. (1992) Dorsal rhizotomy as a treatment for improving function in children with cerebral palsy. In *Movement Disorders in Children* (eds H. Forssberg & H. Hirschfeld), p. 247. Karger, Basel.

Goff, B. (1969) Appropriate afferent stimulation. *Physiotherapy*, **55**, 9.

Goff, B. (1972) The application of recent advances in neurophysiology to Miss M.

Rood's concept of neuromuscular facilitation. *Physiotherapy*, **58**, 409.

Goldkamp, O. (1984) Treatment effectiveness in cerebral palsy. *Arch. Phys. Med. Rehab.*, **65**, 232.

Goldschmied, E. (1975) Playing with babies. In *Creative Therapy* (ed. S. Jennings). Pitman, London.

Goodman, M., Rothberg, A.D. & Jacklin, L.A. (1991) 6 year follow up of early physiotherapy intervention in very low birthweight infants. In *Proceedings of the World Confederation of Physical Therapy Congress*, p. 1211. WCPT, London.

Gordon, J. (1987) Assumptions underlying physical therapy intervention: Theoretical and historical perspectives. In *Movement Science: Foundations for Physical Therapy in Rehabilitation* (eds J.H. Carr & R.B. Shepherd), p. 1. Aspen, Rockville, Maryland.

Gordon, N.S. & McKinlay, I.A. (eds) (1986) *Neurologically Handicapped Children: Treatment and Management*. Blackwell Scientific Publications, Oxford.

Greer, J.G. & Wethered, C.E. (1984) Learned helplessness: a piece of the burnout puzzle. *Exceptional Children*, **50**, 524.

Grenier, A. (1973a) Small walking splint for cerebral palsy children. *CDI Cahiers*, English edition, No. 2. Masson et Cie, Paris.

Grenier, A. (1973b) Pes Valgoplanus in cerebral palsy. The therapeutic role of special shoes for cerebral palsy children. *CDI Cahiers*, English edition, No. 1. Masson et Cié, Paris.

Griffiths, M. & Clegg, M. (1988) *Cerebral Palsy: Problems and Practice*, Chapter 3. Souvenir Press, London.

Griffiths, R. (1967) *The Abilities of Babies*, 4th edn. University of London Press, London.

de Groot, L. (1993) *Posture and Motility in Preterm Infants: A clinical approach*. VU University Press, Amsterdam.

Hagbarth, K.-E. & Eklund, G. (1969) The muscle vibrator – a useful tool in neurological therapeutic work. *Scan. J. Rehab. Med.*, **1**, 26.

Hagberg, B., Hagberg, G. & Olow, I. (1984) The changing panorama of cerebral palsy in Sweden. *Acta Paediatr. Scand.*, **73**, 433.

Hall, D.M.B. (1984) *The Child with a Handicap*. Blackwell Scientific Publications, Oxford.

Hanzlik, J. (1990) Nonverbal interaction patterns of mothers and their infants with cerebral palsy. *Educ. Train. Mental Retard.*, **25**, 333.

Hari, M. & Akos, K. (1990) *Conductive Education*. Routledge, London.

Hari, M. & Tillemans, T. (1984) Conductive education. In *Management of the Motor Disorders of Children with Cerebral Palsy* (ed. D. Scrutton), p. 19. SIMP, Blackwell Scientific Publications, Oxford.

Held, R. (1965) Plasticity in sensory motor systems. *Sci. Am.*, **213**(5), 84.

Hinojosa, J. (1990) How mothers of pre-school children with cerebral palsy perceive occupational and physical therapists and their influence on family life. *Occup. Ther. J. Res.*, **10**, 144.

Hirschfeld, H. (1992) Postural control: acquisition and integration during development. In *Movement Disorders in Children* (eds H. Forssberg & H. Hirschfeld), p. 199. Karger, Basel.

von Hofsten, C. (1992) Development of manual actions from a perceptual perspective. In *Movement Disorders in Children* (eds H. Forssberg & H. Hirschfeld), p. 113. Karger, Basel.

von Hofsten, C. & Ronnqvist, L. (1988) Preparation for grasping an object: a developmental study. *J. Exp. Psychol.*, **4**, 610.

von Hofsten, C. & Rosblad, B. (1988) The integration of sensory information in the development of precise manual pointing. *Neuropsychologia*, **20**, 461.

Holt, K.S. (1965) *Assessment of Cerebral Palsy*, Vol. 1. Lloyd-Luke, London.

Holt, K.S. (1966) Facts and fallacies about neuromuscular function in cerebral palsy as revealed by electromyography. *Dev. Med. Child Neurol.*, **8**, 255.

Holt, K.S. (1973) Discussion of Equinus in *CDI Cahiers*, English edition, No. 1. Masson et Cie, Paris.

Holt, K.S. (ed.) (1975) *Movement and Child Development*, chapters by Holt; Rosenbloom; Wyke; Brand & Rosenbaum; Rosenbaum, Barnitt & Brand; Rosenbloom & Horton. Heinemann – Spastics International Medical Publications, London.

Holt, K.S., Jones, R.B. & Wilson, R. (1974) Gait analysis by means of a multiple sequential camera. *Dev. Med. Child Neurol.*, **16**, 742.

Horak, F.B. (1992) Motor control models underlying neurologic rehabilitation of posture in children. In *Movement Disorders in Children* (eds H. Forssberg & H. Hirschfeld), p. 21. Karger, Basel.

Illingworth, R.S. (1975) *Basic Developmental Screening 0–2 years*. Blackwell Scientific Publications, Oxford.

Illingworth, R.S. (1980) *The Development of the Infant and Young Child, Normal and Abnormal*, 7th edn. Livingstone, Edinburgh and London.

Jacobson, E. (1938) *Progressive Relaxation*. University of Chicago Press.

Jan, J.E., Freeman, R.D. & Scott, E.P. (1977) *Visual Impairment in Children and Adolescents*. Grune & Stratton, New York.

Jones, M. (1993) Serial splinting in hemiplegic cerebral palsy. In *Elements of Paediatric Physiotherapy* (ed. P.M. Eckersley), p. 364. Churchill Livingstone, Edinburgh.

Jones, R.B. (1975) The Vojta method of treatment of cerebral palsy. *Physiotherapy*, **61**, 112.

Kabat, H. (1961) Proprioceptive facilitation in therapeutic exercise. In *Therapeutic Exercise* (ed. S. Licht), 2nd edn, Chapter 13. Licht, New Haven, Connecticut.

Kabat, H., McLeod, M. & Holt, C. (1959) The practical application of Proprioceptive Neuromuscular Facilitation. *Physiotherapy*, **45**, 87.

Kerr, G. (1992) Book review. *Physiotherapy Theory & Practice*, **8**, 127.

Kitzinger, M. (1980) Planning management of feeding in the visually handicapped child. *Child: Care, Health and Development*, **6**, 291.

Knott, M. & Voss, D.E. (1968) *Proprioceptive Neuromuscular Facilitation. Patterns and Techniques*, 2nd edn. Harper & Row, New York.

Knowles, M. (1984) *The Adult Learner: A Neglected Species* (3rd edn). Gulf, Houston.

Kogan, K., Tyler, N. & Turner, P. (1974) The process of interpersonal adaptation between mothers and their cerebral palsied children. *Dev. Med. Child Neurol.*, **16**, 518.

Kong, E. (1987) The importance of early treatment. In *Early Detection and Management of Cerebral Palsy* (eds H. Galjaard, H.F.R. Prechtl & M. Velickovic), p. 107. Martinus Nijhoff, Dordrecht.

Latham, C. (1984) Communicating with children. In *Paediatric Developmental Therapy* (ed. S. Levitt). Blackwell Scientific Publications, Oxford.

Leach, M. (1993) *Activities for People with a Multiple Disability*. The Spastics Society, London.

Leonard, C.T., Hirschfeld, H. & Forssberg, H. (1988) Gait acquisition and reflex abnormalities in normal children and children with cerebral palsy. In *Posture and Gait: Development, Adaptation and Modulation* (eds B. Amblard, A. Berthoz & F. Clarac), p. 33. Elsevier, Amsterdam.

Leonard, C.T., Hirschfeld, H. & Forssberg, H. (1991) The development of independent walking in children with cerebral palsy. *Dev. Med. Child Neurol.*, **33**, 567.

Levitt, S. (1962) *Physiotherapy in Cerebral Palsy*. Thomas, Springfield, Illinois.

Levitt, S. (1966) Proprioceptive Neuromuscular Facilitation techniques in cerebral palsy. *Physiotherapy*, **52**, 46.

Levitt, S. (1967) Motor behaviour in cerebral palsy and relevant proprioceptive neuromuscular facilitation techniques. *Sjukgymnasten*, November.

Levitt, S. (1969a) Relaxation in cerebral palsy (selection of methods from various systems). Paper published in *Proceedings of the International Symposium on the Disabled Child in Bruges, Belgium, September 1969.*

Levitt, S. (1969b) *Cerebral Palsy and the Young Child* (ed. S. Blencowe), Chapter 7. Livingstone, London.

Levitt, S. (1969c) The treatment of cerebral palsy and proprioceptive neuromuscular facilitation techniques. In *On the Treatment of Spastic Pareses*. Institute Neurology, Stockholm. *Sjukgymnasten*, **27**, 3.

Levitt, S. (1970a) Principles of treatment in cerebral palsy. *Fysioterapeuten*, **10**.

Levitt, S. (1970b) Adaptation of PNF for cerebral palsy. In *Proceedings of the World Confederation of Physical Therapy Congress, Amsterdam*. WCPT, London.

Levitt, S. (1974) Common factors in the different systems of treatment in cerebral palsy. *CDI Cahiers*, No. 59, Masson et Cie, Paris.

Levitt, S. (1976) Stimulation of movement: A review of therapeutic techniques. In *Early Management of Handicapping Disorders* (eds T.E. Oppé & F.P. Woodford). IRMMH. Associated Scientific Publishers, Amsterdam, reprinted from *Movement and Child Development* (ed. K.S. Holt), Heinemann – Spastics International Medical Publications, London.

Levitt, S. (1982) Movement training. In *Profound Mental Handicap* (ed. D. Norris). Costello, Tunbridge Wells.

Levitt, S. (ed.) (1984) *Paediatric Developmental Therapy*. Blackwell Scientific Publications, Oxford.

Levitt, S. (1986) Handling the child with paediatric developmental disability. *Physiotherapy*, **72**, 161.

Levitt, S. (1987) Therapy for the motor disorders. In *Early Detection and Management of Cerebral Palsy* (eds H. Galjaard, H.F.R. Prechtl & M. Velickovic), p. 113. Martinus Nijhoff, Dordrecht.

Levitt, S. (1991) International therapy workshops. In *Proceedings of the 11th International Congress of the WCPT*, p. 283. WCPT, London.

Levitt, S. (1994) *Basic Abilities – A Whole Approach*. Souvenir Press, London.

Levitt, S. & Goldschmied, E. (1990) As we teach, so we treat. *Physiotherapy Theory & Practice*, **6**, 227.

Levitt, S. & Miller, C. (1973) The interrelationships of speech therapy and physiotherapy in children with neurodevelopmental disorders. *Dev. Med. Child Neurol.*, **15**, 2.

McCarthy G.T. (ed.) (1992) *The Physically Handicapped Child*, 2nd edn. Faber & Faber, London.

McConachie, H. (1986) Parents' contribution to the education of their child. In *The Education of Children with Severe Learning Difficulties: Bridging the Gap between Theory and Practice* (eds J. Coupe & J. Porter), p. 253. Croom Helm, London.

McGraw, M. (1966) *The Neuromuscular Maturation of the Human Infant*. Hafner, New York.

McKinlay, I.A. (1989) Therapy for cerebral palsy. *Seminars Orthopaed.*, **4**, 220.

McKinlay, I.A., Hyde, E. & Gordon, N.S. (1980) Baclofen: a team approach to drug evaluation of spasticity in childhood. In *Baclofen: A Broader Spectrum of Activity*, p. 26. A supplement to *Scott. Med. J.*

McLellan, L. (1984) Therapeutic possibilities in cerebral palsy: a neurologist's view. In *Management of the Motor Disorders of Children with Cerebral Palsy* (ed. D. Scrutton), p. 96. SIMP, Blackwell Scientific Publications, Oxford.

Marsden, C.D., Merton, P.A. & Merton, H.B. (1981) Human postural responses. *Brain*, **104**, 513.

Martin, J.P. (1965) Tilting reactions and disorders of the basal ganglia. *Brain*, **88**, 855.

Martin, J.P. (1967) *The Basal Ganglia and Posture*. Pitman Medical Publications, London.

Milani-Comparetti, A. & Gidoni, E.A. (1967) Routine developmental examination in normal and retarded children. *Dev. Med. Child Neurol.*, **9**, 625.

Miller, C.J. (1972) The speech therapist and the group treatment of young cerebral palsied children. *Br. J. Disord. Commun.* 7, No. 2.

Mitchell, R.G. (1977) The nature and causes of disability in childhood. In *Neurodevelopmental Problems in Early Childhood: Assessment and Management* (eds C.M. Drillien & M.B. Drummond), Chapter 1. Blackwell Scientific Publications, Oxford.

Morgenstern, M., Low-Beer, H. & Morgenstern, F. (1966) *Practical Training for the Severely Handicapped Child*. Heinemann, London.

Mulcahy, C.M., Pountney, T.E., Nelham, R.L., Green, E.M. & Billington, G.D. (1988) Adaptive seating for motor handicap: problems, a solution, assessment and prescription. *Br. J. Occup. Ther.*, **51**, 347.

Mulder, T. (1985) *The Learning of Motor Control Following Brain Damage: Experimental and Clinical Studies*. Swets & Zeitlinger, Lisse.

Mulder, T. (1991) A process oriented model of human motor behavior: implications for rehabilitation medicine. *Phy. Ther.*, **71**, 157.

Mulder, T. & Hulstijn, W. (1988) From movement to action: The learning of motor control following brain damage. In *Complex Human Movement Behavior* (eds O.G. Meijer & K. Roth), p. 247. Elsevier, Amsterdam.

Myhr, U. & von Wendt, L. (1990) Reducing spasticity and enhancing postural control for the creation of a functional sitting position in children with cerebral palsy: A pilot study. *Physiotherapy Theory & Practice*, **6**, 65.

Nashner, L.M., Shumway-Cook, A. & Marin, O. (1983) Stance posture in select groups of children with cerebral palsy: deficits in sensory organisation and muscular condition. *Exp. Brain Res.*, **49**, 393.

Nathan, P. (1969) Annotation: treatment of spasticity with peri-neural injections of phenol. *Dev. Med. Child Neurol.*, **11**, 384.

Nelson, K.B. & Ellenberg, J.H. (1982) Children who 'outgrew' cerebral palsy. *Pediatrics*, **69**, 529.

Neumann Neurodde, D. (1967) *Baby Gymnastics*. Pergamon Press, London & Oxford.

Newson, E. (1976) Parents as a resource in diagnosis and assessment. In *Early Management of Handicapping Disorders* (eds T.E. Oppé & F.P. Woodford), p. 105. Associated Scientific Publishers, Amsterdam.

Norén, L. & Franzén, G. (1982) An evaluation of 7 postural reactions selected by Vojta in 25 healthy infants. *Neuropediatrics*, **12**, 308.

Nwaobi, O.M. (1987) Seating orientations and upper extremity function in children with cerebral palsy. *Phys. Ther.*, **67**, 1209.

Nwaobi, O.M., Brubaker, C., *et al.* (1983) Electromyographic investigation of extensor activity in cerebral palsy children in different seating positions. *Dev. Med. Child Neurol.*, **25**, 175.

Olow, I. (1986) Children with cerebral palsy. In *Neurologically Handicapped Children: Treatment and management* (eds N.S. Gordon & I.A. McKinlay), p. 60. Blackwell Scientific Publications, Oxford.

Oppenheim, R.W. (1981) Ontogenetic adaptations and retrogressive processes in the development of the nervous system and behavior: A neuro-embryological perspective. In *Maturation and Development* (eds K.J. Connolly & H.F.R. Prechtl), p. 73. Heinemann, London.

Paine, R.S. (1964) The evolution of infantile postural reflexes in the presence of chronic brain syndromes. *Dev. Med. Child Neurol.*, **6**, 345.

Paine, R.S. & Oppé, T.E. (1966) *Neurological Examination of Children.* Heinemann Books – Spastics International Medical Publications, London.

Palmer, F.B., Shapiro, B.K., Wachtel, R.C., *et al.* (1988) The effects of physical therapy on cerebral palsy. *N. Engl. J. Med.,* **318**, 803.

Parette, H.P. & Hourcade, J.J. (1984) A review of therapeutic intervention research on gross and fine motor progress in young children with cerebral palsy. *Am. J. Occup. Ther.,* **38**, 462.

Pearson, P.H. & Williams, C.E. (eds) (1972) *Physical Therapy Services in the Developmental Disabilities.* Thomas, Springfield, Illinois.

Pederson, E. (1969) *Spasticity, Mechanism, Measurement, Management.* Thomas, Springfield, Illinois.

Peiper, A. (1963) *Cerebral Function in Infancy and Childhood.* Consultants Bureau, New York. Also Pitman Medical, London.

Penso, D.E. (1987) *Occupational Therapy for Children with Disabilities.* Croom Helm, London.

Phelps, W.M. (1949) Description and differentiation of types of cerebral palsy. *Nerv. Child,* **8**, 107.

Phelps, W.M. (1952) The rôle of physical therapy in cerebral palsy and bracing in the cerebral palsies. In *Orthopaedic Appliances Atlas 1*, pp. 251–522. Edwards, Ann Arbor.

Plum, P. & Molhave, A. (1956) Clinical analysis of static and dynamic patterns in cerebral palsy with a view to active correction. *Arch. Phys. Med.,* **37**, 8.

Prechtl, H.F.R. (1977) *The Neurological Examination of the Full Term Newborn Infant.* Clin. Dev. Med., No. 63. SIMP–Heinemann, London.

Prechtl, H.F.R. (1981) The study of neural development as prospective of clinical problems. In *Maturation and Development* (eds K.J. Connolly & H.F.R. Prechtl). Heinemann, London.

Presland, J.L. (1982) *Paths to Mobility in 'Special Care'*, pp. 19, 35–8. British Institute of Mental Handicap, Kidderminster.

Price, E., Thylefors, I. & von Wendt, L. (1991) The role of the physiotherapist in the Swedish paediatric rehabititation teams. In *Proceedings of the World Confederation of Physical Therapy Congress, London*, p. 1187. WCPT, London.

Reynell, J. & Zinkin, P. (1975) New procedures for the developmental assessment of young children with severe visual handicaps. *Child: Care, Health and Development,* **1**, 61.

Riddoch, J. & Lennon, S. (1991) Evaluation of practice: The single case study approach. *Physiotherapy Theory & Practice,* **7**, 3.

Roberts, D.M. (1978) *Neurophysiology of Postural Mechanisms,* 2nd edn. Butterworth, London.

Robson, P. (1970) Shuffling, hitching, scooting or sliding: some observations in 30 otherwise normal children. *Dev. Med. Child. Neurol.,* **12**, 608.

Rogers, C. (1983) *Freedom to Learn for the 80s.* Merrill, Columbus, Ohio.

Rood, M.S. (1956) Neurophysiological mechanisms utilized in the treatment of neuromuscular dysfunction. *Am. J. Occup. Ther.,* **10**(4) part 2, 220.

Rood, M.S. (1962) Use of sensory receptors to activate, facilitate and inhibit motor response, automatic and somatic, in developmental sequence. In *Approaches to the Treatment of Patients with Neuromuscular Dysfunction* (ed. C. Sattely). *Third International Congress of World Federation of Occupational Therapists.*

Rosblad, B. & von Hofsten, C. (1992) Perceptual control of manual pointing in children with motor impairments. *Physiotherapy Theory & Practice,* **8**, 223.

Rosenbaum, P.L., King, S.M. & Cadman, D.T. (1992) Measuring processes of caregiving to physically disabled children and their families I: Identifying relevant components of care. *Dev. Med. Child Neurol.,* **34**, 103.

Ross, K. & Thomson, D. (1993) An evaluation of parents' involvement in the management of their cerebral palsy children. *Physiotherapy,* **79**, 561.